The Yoga of Pregnancy

The Yoga of

CONNECT WITH YOUR UNBORN CHILD
THROUGH YOUR MIND, BODY AND BREATH

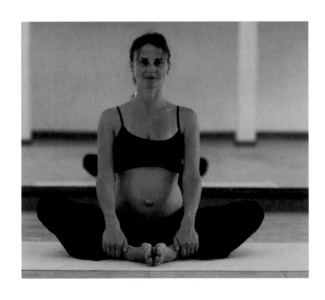

Pregnancy

A 40-week journey of narrations, intentions, meditations, affirmations and yoga to help you connect with your unborn baby

MEL CAMPBELL

FINDHORN PRESS

Published in 2012 by Findhorn Press, Scotland

ISBN 978-1-84409-593-3

Photos by Ryan Libre, Documentary Arts Asia © 2008
Matt Campbell © 2012 (p. 6–7.)
Michael Mitton © 2012 (pp. 18, 34, 38, 58, 74, 88, 94, 110, 120, 130, 142–3, 144)

Edited by Jacqui Lewis
Cover design by Damian Keenan
Designed in Kingfisher by Geoff Green Book Design
Printed and bound in the EU

1 2 3 4 5 6 7 8 9 17 16 15 14 13 12

Published by
Findhorn Press
117–121 High Street
Forres IV36 1AB
Scotland, UK

t +44 (0)1309 690582
f +44 (0)131 777 2711

e info@findhornpress.com
www.findhornpress.com

Disclaimer

The information in this book is given in good faith and is neither
intended to diagnose any physical or mental condition nor to serve
as a substitute for informed medical advice or care.
Please contact your health professional for medical advice and
treatment. Neither author nor publisher can be held liable by any
person for any loss or damage whatsoever which may arise from the
use of this book or any of the information therein.

To my three beautiful daughters
Esmé, Phoebe and Evi

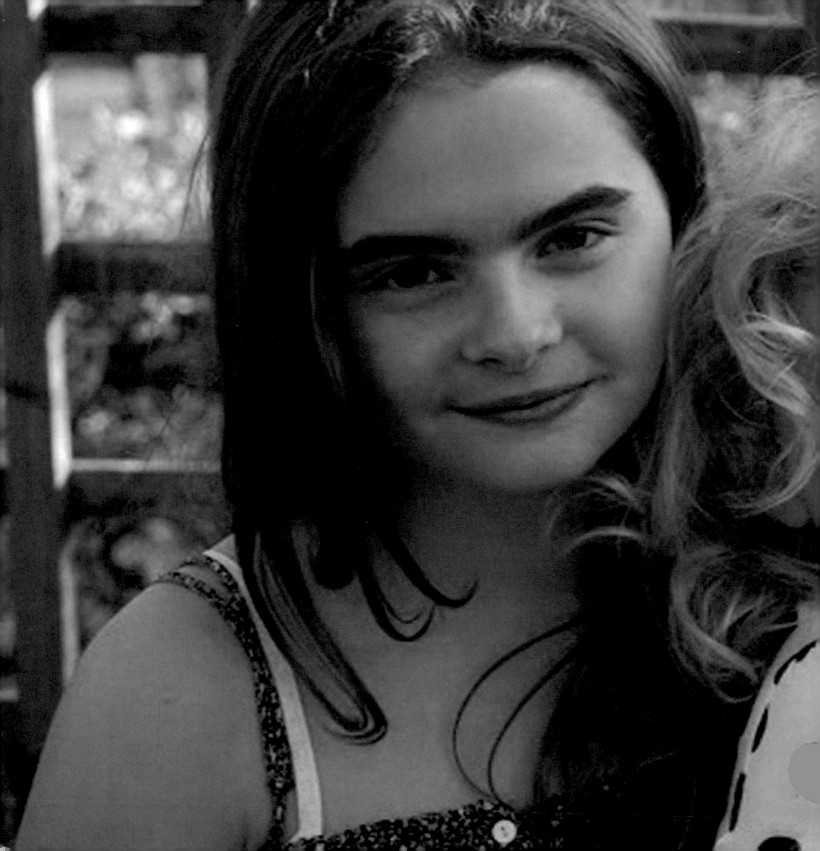

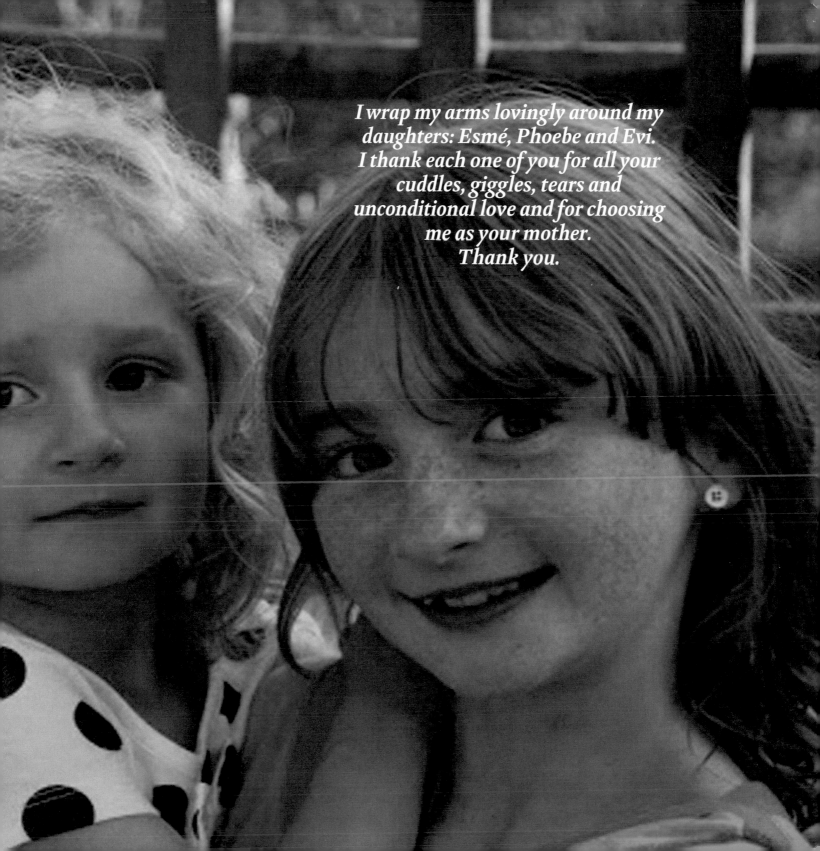

*I wrap my arms lovingly around my
daughters: Esmé, Phoebe and Evi.
I thank each one of you for all your
cuddles, giggles, tears and
unconditional love and for choosing
me as your mother.
Thank you.*

Acknowledgements

I found a comfortable seat, I rested my hands around my bump and cradled you. I closed my eyes and marged with the rhythm of my breath. I connected with you through my mind, body and breath and together we practised **The Yoga of Pregnancy***. Thank-you Evi, for sharing my practice with me and for being my inspiration for this book.*

Thank you to my husband Matt, who was privileged to encounter all the hormones released throughout each one of my trimesters during each of my pregnancies, and throughout the writing of this book. Thank you for your forever-endearing love, support, encouragement and for sharing all of my dreams.

I would also like to share my gratitude to The Yoga Studio, Chiang Mai, Jennifer Van Der Park for her assistance and sharp eye during the photoshoot, and to Ryan Libre for his ongoing patience with this project.

I would like to thank all my yoga teachers, who have shared their wisdom and gifts with me over the years, and all my students, who continually inspire me.

Finally, I would like to thank Findhorn Press for believing in my project and to my editors Sabine and Jacqui for their clarity, commitment, time and vision during the delivery of this book and for helping me to realize my dream.

The light within me bows to and honors the light within each and every one of you.

NAMASTÉ

This book is aimed at mothers-to-be who wish to celebrate pregnancy and explore the joy of prenatal yoga.

If you are feeling fatigued during your pregnancy yet still wish to practise yoga asanas (poses), please respect your body and refer to the restorative poses or pranayama (breath) exercises in this book that are indicated as being suitable for your trimester.

Remember that your body is changing and may feel different every day and that each pregnancy is a unique experience, even for the same woman. If something doesn't feel comfortable in your practice, the rule is: don't do it. If it is uncomfortable for you to hold any pose for the length of breaths indicated, please rest in an appropriate pose such as Child's Pose and return to the pose only when you feel ready.

The hormone relaxin is released during your pregnancy to help stretch your ligaments and connective tissues to open your body and prepare it for labor. It is not uncommon for women to experience discomfort in the pelvic girdle due to the increased mobility in the pelvic joints.

It is advised that you bear in mind this increased flexibility and take care not to over-stretch your body when practising asanas, or when doing any other form of exercise.

To minimize the risk of pelvic discomfort or damage, it is recommended that you avoid deep squats and asymmetrical poses and always refer to the notes of caution provided.

Before you begin the course of yoga outlined in this book, familiarize yourself with the poses and ensure that you have everything you need: any yoga props you may want to use, drinking water, soothing music if you like. Wear comfortable loose clothing and remember to allow one to two hours after eating before you start a yoga practice or any other exercise.

If you have never practised yoga before, you are advised to seek out a certified prenatal yoga instructor and attend classes specifically designed for pregnancy, and to use this book only as an additional source of guidance.

Please consult your doctor or midwife before attempting any of the poses or other practices in this book. The reader assumes their own responsibility and the author is not responsible for any injuries incurred.

Please note: The author was photographed for the purpose of this book during her second and third trimester of pregnancy; therefore the photographs are not an accurate representation of each week of pregnancy.

Contents

Introduction

Yoga is the Sanskrit word for "union", and through the practice of yoga the mind, body and breath are united.

During pregnancy you live and breathe with your baby and he or she becomes aware of your thoughts, movements and emotions; so it seems only natural that they should be included in your yoga practice.

Each chapter of this book honors the weekly development and physiological changes taking place within both you and your growing baby. These changes are reflected and supported by the practices of affirmation, meditation, pranayama (breathing techniques) and asana (poses) to help you unite with your baby through your mind, body and breath. By deepening your awareness of your growing baby in this way, you can enhance and embrace all the stages of your pregnancy and prepare yourself mentally, physically and emotionally for labor, giving birth, and motherhood.

The first trimester of a pregnancy is the most challenging in terms of practising yoga. Although there is usually no visible evidence of the pregnancy, on the inside your body is going through rapid, daily changes. As your baby starts to make its home in your uterus, it develops from a single embryonic cell into a growing fetus. The physical make-up of your growing baby is formed by the end of week nine, and by the end of the first trimester it is moving effortlessly around in its oceanic sea of amniotic fluid.

During these first 12 weeks, it is vital that you listen carefully to your body, letting the body's innate wisdom be your guide and respecting any cues it may give you. Pregnancy is not the time to overexert yourself; rather, it is a time to relinquish any temptations to overachieve and to focus instead on a mindful practice of meditation, pranayama and restorative yoga poses that honors both your changing body and your growing baby.

As you enter the second trimester, you will hopefully feel more energized; this is the period when nausea, morning sickness and tiredness usually abate.

The intention or aim for this stage of your pregnancy is to help prepare you to give birth. In this book the focus of the practice at this point is on standing postures, squats and hip openers. These will help to build stamina, increase strength in your thighs and create freedom in the hips and around the pelvis, to help prepare you physically for giving birth.

During the final months of pregnancy, you are encouraged to conserve your energy and return to a practice of restorative yoga, meditation, visualizations and positive thinking. You are invited to replace any fears you may have about labor and the impending birth of your child with positive thoughts (affirmations) and visualizations. These practices will help you to mentally prepare yourself for labor and the delivery of your child, encouraging you to focus on and develop qualities such as courage, patience, acceptance and trust as you focus on having a labor of love and a happy birth-day.

Breath techniques are particularly focused on during this trimester, as they are very useful in supporting you during labor and delivery.

The hormones released during the birthing process are those designed to make you feel euphoric. If you can develop the ability to listen to your instincts, trust, have faith and surrender to the occasion, this, combined with the cumulative effects and habits of practising yoga and meditation throughout your pregnancy, can all combine to make giving birth a spiritual as well as a physical and mental experience.

By gently moving and exercising your body in an asana practice, you can become more aware of the needs of your body and your baby. You can learn to listen to and trust your intuition, and prepare your body physically for the demands of labor, so that your body is open and ready to receive the birth of your baby with grace.

By meditating on your breath, using different breath techniques and incorporating sound into your practice, you can become more familiar with the capacity your body has to naturally release tension and ease discomfort.

By bonding and uniting with your unborn child through the practice of affirmations, intentions and visualizations, you can prepare yourself emotionally and spiritually, tuning in to and developing your inherent maternal instincts.

These are the lessons you can learn and the gifts you can receive as you follow your yoga practice during your pregnancy, to take with you into labor, birth and on into motherhood. This book is an invitation to you to find, feel and experience your own yoga of pregnancy.

So I invite you to thumb through the pages, curl over the edges, scribble in the corners, cry, laugh, love and enjoy giving birth to your own practice.

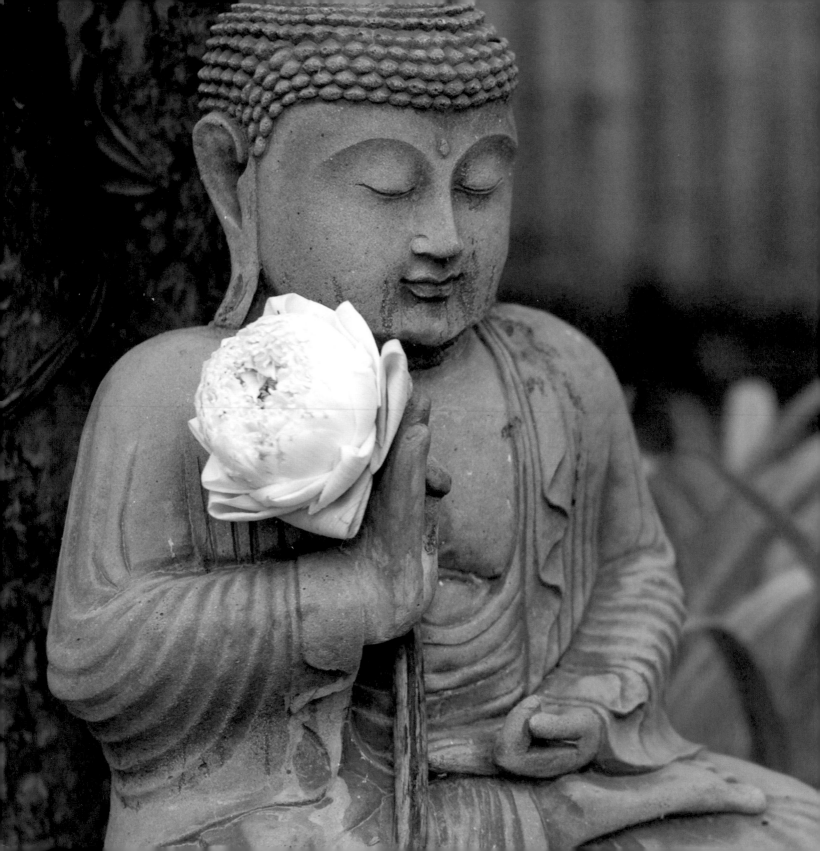

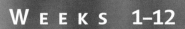

The First Trimester

In the first trimester of my pregnancy I will unite with my baby through practices of meditation and gentle yoga that honor the rapid changes taking place in my body during these early months.

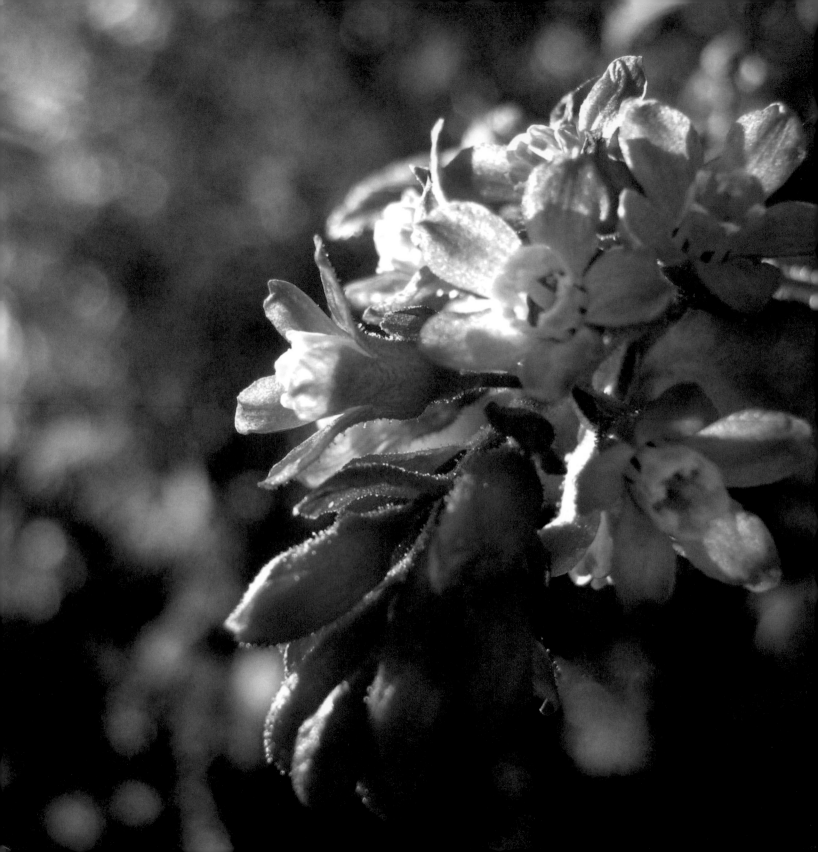

Our New Beginnings

I am fully prepared and committed to welcome this new life,
as my growing baby begins to develop inside of me.

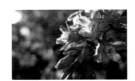

This week I will rest my body, relax my mind and befriend my breath, uniting with you in honor of our new beginnings.

A little blue line confirmed for me you are here.

Just a few tiny cells for now, the size of an apple seed, you are busy nestling into my uterus, where you will soon find a home to settle and grow over the next forty weeks.

Although I am barely pregnant, I nevertheless find myself naturally protecting you with my hands as you begin your quest for life.

I am excited yet nervous, knowing that over just forty weeks you will grow from some tiny cells not yet visible to the naked eye into my beautiful baby, who I will mother.

The signs of you being here are already beginning to show; my tastes are changing, smells are enhanced, my breasts are tender, and feelings of nausea and fatigue are emerging.

I try to welcome them all, in the knowledge that we both have an incredible journey of physical, emotional and spiritual growth and change ahead of us.

Intention

This week I will pack my imaginary bag for my new life ahead of me. I shall think about all the things I would like to take with me to enhance my experience:

courage, wisdom, faith, acceptance;

and choose what I would like to leave behind:

fear, anxiety, worries, concerns.

I will make friends with my inner self, who I will be traveling with, and greet her with love, laughter and joy.

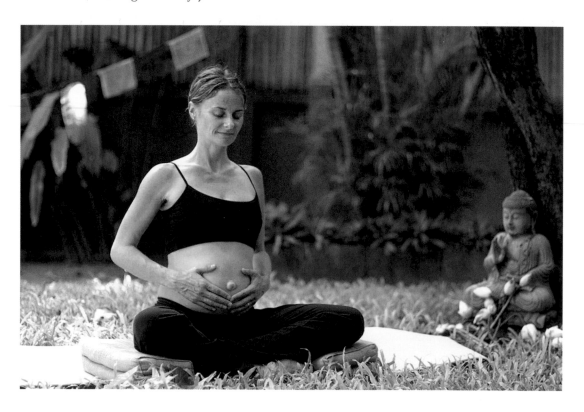

Pranayama for the Week

Abdominal Breathing

For this practice I will need a yoga mat and a small cushion.

   This exercise is suitable for all stages of my pregnancy.

❋ I find a comfortable cross-legged sitting position and bring my hands around my belly.

❋ I close my eyes and take a moment to welcome you into my life. I find the natural rhythm of my breath and ride on the waves of my breath coming and going.

❋ Deepening my inhalations and lengthening my exhalations, I direct my breath down to you.

❋ I notice my belly rising when I inhale and falling when I exhale.

❋ This is abdominal breathing.

❋ I keep my breaths smooth and steady, being mindful of your presence.

❋ Staying connected with my breath for several minutes, I mindfully repeat this week's affirmation:

I am fully prepared and committed to welcome this new life,
as my growing baby begins to develop inside of me.

BENEFITS: Abdominal Breathing improves circulation and respiration; soothes the nervous system; focuses and calms the mind.

CAUTIONS: If I have pelvic girdle discomfort I will practise this breath sitting on my heels with my knees together. I will place a cushion(s) between my sitting bones and my heels to bridge any gaps.

Reflection

In union we found peace in our body and mind,
finding a foundation from which to begin the journey of
our new beginnings.

NAMASTÉ

WEEK 7

Our Union of Hearts

My baby is an expression of my love I have to share.

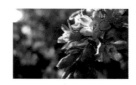

BENEFITS: *Heart Opener Pose strengthens the front of the thighs and ankles; lengthens the spine; opens the shoulders and the chest.*

CAUTIONS: *In my second trimester, as my uterus stretches to accommodate my growing baby I will be careful not to overstretch the front of my body in this pose and only practise the first stage of this pose if it continues to feel comfortable, I will avoid this pose if I have any knee issues.*

MODIFICATIONS: *If I feel in the full pose any discomfort in my lower back, or too much of a deep stretch in my abdominal area, I will practise the first stage only.*

This week I will open my heart, connecting the rhythm of my soul with your new heartbeat in our union of hearts.

Already you have grown to the size of a grape.

This week your major organs – brain, spinal cord, kidneys, lungs, pancreas, kidneys, liver, heart – are being mapped out, with the major roads of your larger blood vessels being defined. Your simple heart begins to function, pumping the fluid through these blood vessels, creating its own unique rhythm, regularly pulsating.

Inside my body remarkable changes are taking place.

There is a shift in my hormone levels as you begin to grow and your placenta develops, making me feel tired, highly sensitive and emotional.

I am aware that the vibration of my heart has an effect on your heart, so I am trying to stay calm amongst all these changes.

I remind myself to tenderly rest my hands on my belly, to connect to my center and unite myself with you, imagining that with each beat of my heart my love resounds in yours.

Intention

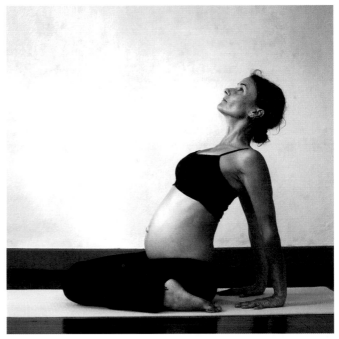

As I rest my hands over my heart and close my eyes,
I will check in on the weather of my heart.
How am I feeling today?
Feeling my heartbeat from the inside out, I will simply stay a
while, listening to its own unique rhythmical beat.
I will think of all the people who love and support me in my
life, I will think of all the people whom I love,
and I will think of you.

Asana for the Week

Heart Opener Pose

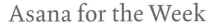

For this pose I will need a yoga mat.

This pose is suitable for the first two trimesters of my pregnancy.

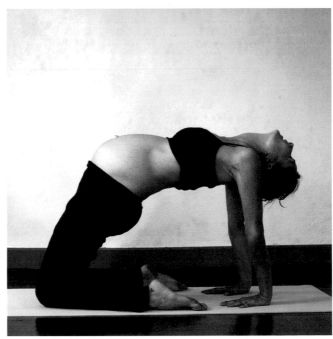

- I come onto all fours into a tabletop position. I slide my legs outwards, one to each side, and carefully sit down in between my feet. I place my hands on the floor behind me with my fingers facing forward.

- I roll my shoulders down and back and breathe into my upper chest. I feel my heart open and lift up towards the sky.

- Closing my eyes, I stay here for five breaths enjoying the feeling of expansion in my upper chest and my heart center.

- I visualize the path of our love traveling from my love center to yours and from your love center to mine. This is our union of hearts.

- Lifting my hips up, I now come into my full expression of the pose.

- Staying for five breaths, I mindfully repeat this week's affirmation:

    My baby is an expression of my love I have to share.

✦ I release out of the pose, close my eyes and sit for a minute with you.

✦ I notice any changes in my mind, body and breath.

Reflection

Through my practice I opened my heart and connected
the rhythm of my love with yours in
our union of hearts.

NAMASTÉ

The Essence of Being

Each breath I take sends energy to my growing baby.

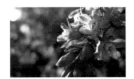

This week I will connect to the rhythm of my breath and celebrate the essence of being.

This week you form the shape of your face.

Like two little dimples your eyes appear, like a delicate soft floret your nose appears with two small impressions ready to form your nostrils, and a little mouth emerges, soon to wear your smile.

Your tiny limbs lengthen and stretch, corresponding to the development of your first joints, the hips, knees, shoulders and elbows. Your curved, arched appearance straightens out a little, as you extend out through them.

Like tiny buds your hands and feet have a fusion of digits, ready to germinate and blossom into feeling fingers and touching toes.

Sporadically your new nervous system practises sending messages through your body, causing you to move and jerk in an uncoordinated fashion. It will, though, still be several weeks before I feel you move inside me.

BENEFITS: *Utkata Konasana Flow opens the hips and the groin area; improves circulation and calms the mind.*

CAUTIONS: *If I have pelvic girdle discomfort I will take a narrower stance by bringing my feet apart only as wide as my outer hips. It is advised that I do not practise deep or unsupported squats after week 34 of my pregnancy or once my baby is engaged.*

MODIFICATIONS: *To practise this pose in a supported squat I sit on several cushions and bend my knees, as demonstrated on page 40. I check to ensure that my hips are slightly higher than my knees, and if they are not I use extra cushions to sit a little higher. My feet are firmly grounded on the floor. I follow the movements of my hands, flowing through the practice while I remain seated in a supported squat position.*

Intention

As I wrap my arms around my belly,
I shall think of how your tiny joints are evolving
and you begin to move for the very first time.
As I go about my daily life this week,
I will fully appreciate each movement my body makes,
imagining I am creating it for the very first time.

Asana for the Week

Utkata Konasana Flow – The Goddess Flow

For this pose I will need a yoga mat.

    This pose is suitable for all three trimesters (although see 'Cautions', left).

❀ Taking a wide stance along my yoga mat with my feet facing forward and parallel to each other, I turn my feet out at a slight angle, making sure my heels are in line with each other.

❀ I bend my knees, stacking them directly above my ankles and ensuring that they are aligned with my second and third toes.

❀ I bring my hands to form a shape like an opening flower in front of my heart center; the outside edges of my little fingers and the inside edges of my thumbs touch, and the heels of my hands stay connected (a).

❀ I tenderly look at my hands and take a breath. I see you as my budding flower and I send nutrients and nourishment to you through my body and breath.

❀ Inhaling, I raise my hands above my head; I follow their movements with my eyes. Simultaneously I straighten my legs (b).

❀ Exhaling, I curl my fingers over, so the backs of the fingers touch each other. Softly I bend my knees and lower my arms (c).

❀ Once again I form the shape of an opening flower with my hands and rest them in front of my heart (a).

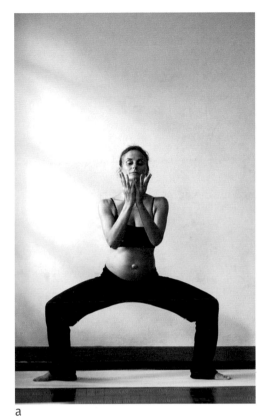
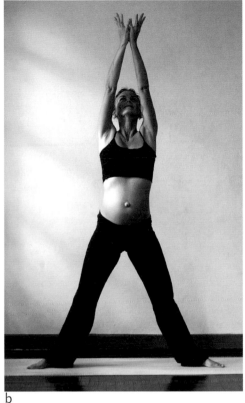
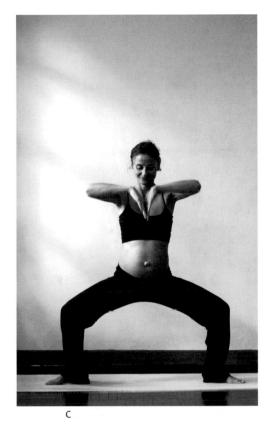

a   b   c

✿ Repeating this flow five times, I synchronize the movements with my breath.

✿ Mindfully I repeat this week's affirmation:

Each breath I take sends energy to my growing baby.

Reflection

This week I invited softness into my physical body,
a sense of peace within my mind and openness within my heart.
Synchronizing my movements with my breath I enjoyed
the essence of being.

NAMASTÉ

WEEK 9

Nurturing and Nourishing

As I nurture my body, my body nourishes my growing baby.

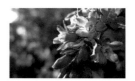

During my pregnancy it is vital I stay healthy in my mind, body and spirit, maintaining my well-being so I can support my growing baby in ways which are equally nourishing and nurturing.

You are so tiny, about an inch in length, yet your physical framework is more or less formed already. You even have arms, legs, a torso and a head, and some of your rudimentary muscles and organs have even started their preliminary functions.

Unconsciously you begin to move as your major muscular system starts to communicate with your nerves. It is hard to believe that you are still so tiny, yet you are moving around independently, twisting, turning, like a graceful dancer suspended in your ocean of amniotic fluid.

The muscle of your heart is working hard, beating twice as fast as that of an adult. Soon I will have the honor of seeing you and listening to your heartbeat at our first ultrasound visit. This moment will be etched on my memory forever.

At the moment your heart is composed of two love centers, which will soon divide into the four main chambers to support your ever-flowing blood supply.

As you evolve, crafting your more intricate details and functions, my body supports you, adapting to these changes from the inside out.

So while my body cares for you I need to take care of my body, providing me with the perfect excuse to slow down and relax.

Intention

Together we take a moment to find stillness and take a rest.
Together we take a moment to reflect on all we have achieved.
Together we take a moment to be proud.
Together we unite in our hearts, and the beauty of all that we share.
Together we take a moment to enjoy the essence of who we are
and who we are becoming;
a mother; a child.

Asana for the Week

Supported Reclining Pose

For this pose I will need a yoga mat, a bolster or long pillow, a blanket, a small cushion for my head and two more cushions or folded blankets for my arms, and an eye pillow.
  This pose is suitable for all stages of my pregnancy.

❀ I sit on my yoga mat with a short end of a bolster or long pillow against my lower back. I place a small cushion on the other end of the bolster and another cushion, or folded blanket, at each side of the mat where my arms will rest.

❀ Reclining carefully back over the bolster or long pillow, I ensure that my back is comfortably supported, and if it isn't I use my hands to push myself back up, reposition the pillow and recline again. I place a rolled blanket under my knees.

❀ I rest my head on the cushion, so my head is raised slightly higher than my heart center and my heart center is raised slightly higher than you. My upper chest is open, with my forearms softly extending out to the sides, each supported by a cushion.

❀ I close my eyes and place an eye pillow over my eyes.

BENEFITS: Supported Reclining Pose improves breathing and circulation; relieves tension in the shoulders; opens the upper chest; soothes the nervous system and calms the mind.

CAUTIONS: From week 18 on, it is advised that I do not lie flat on my back. To continue to practise this pose later in my pregnancy I can use extra props to support me in a semi-reclined position.
I will stop practising this pose if it becomes uncomfortable for me. I will let my body be my guide.

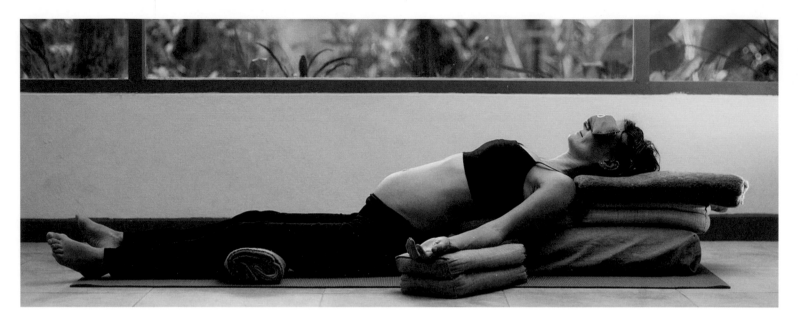

❀ I take a deep sigh and connect with the natural rhythm of my breath.

❀ I relax and surrender into the pose, feeling it nurture and nourish both of our bodies and souls.

❀ Staying here for up to ten minutes, I mindfully repeat this week's affirmation:

As I nurture my body, my body nourishes my growing baby.

❀ Afterwards I remove my eye pillow, bend my knees and roll over to my left side. I stay here for a few minutes before using my hands to gently assist me up into a sitting position.

Reflection

This week, while my body took care of my baby,
I took care of my body, learning to relax in ways which were both
nurturing and nourishing.

NAMASTÉ

Our Spines

The cells of my growing baby are learning to interact with each other to create a union of the body and mind.

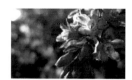

This week we will honor the union of the body and mind in a practice dedicated to our spines.

Congratulations

This week you have reached a new landmark in your incredible journey, emerging from your embryonic stage as you change into a fetus.

Your embryonic tail has disappeared and instinctively you curl up into the fetal position to rest. You bring your knees to your chest, tuck your chin in and allow your spine to softly round and establish its natural curves in this shape.

The complexity of your spine continues to evolve. Nerve cells multiply and form pathways around your body, creating a sophisticated network of connections to your developing brain.

While the labyrinth of your nervous system is being carefully crafted beneath your transparent skin, primary movements are initiated. Spontaneously you begin to fidget, exercising your muscles to stimulate their growth and experiencing ways to move your body.

You have grown so much over the last few weeks, yet still you remain a secret to the outside world.

No sign of a pregnant belly yet; for now, you are my hidden treasure.

Intention

As I twist, turn, stretch, fold, curl and uncurl my spine this week,
I will think of you.
I will imagine your spine and your body moving
from your newly awakened nervous system,
sending ripples of movement through your
ocean of amniotic fluid.

Asana for the Week

Uttanasana – Standing Forward Fold

For this pose I will need a yoga mat.
   This pose is suitable for all stages of my pregnancy.

BENEFITS: *Uttanasana stretches the hamstrings, hips and calves; strengthens the thighs; and calms the mind.*

CAUTIONS: *If I have any lower-back discomfort I will keep my knees bent (c) while practising this pose.*

MODIFICATIONS: *If my spine rounds in this pose or I feel an intense stretch down the back of my legs in (a, b), I will practise with my knees bent (c, d).*

✤ Standing with my feet parallel and outer-hip width apart, I take a forward fold, my spine cascading down like a waterfall.

✤ Each vertebra is soft and flowing in union with its neighbor.

✤ I think of your spine softly curving, finding its natural resting position.

✤ I try to keep my legs straight as I reach down to the floor with my hands. If I can I place them down in front of my feet (a), otherwise I bend my knees (c).

✤ Inhaling, I slide my hands onto the fronts of my calves, lifting and lengthening the front of my body to come up halfway with a straight spine (b or d).

✤ Exhaling, I bow down, bringing my hands to rest on the earth again.

✤ I repeat this three times, thinking of you as I move my spine dynamically, sending ripples through my vertebrae and movements through my body.

✤ On my third exhalation I fold forward for three breaths, mindfully repeating this week's affirmation:

The cells of my growing baby are learning to interact with each
other to create a union of the body and mind.

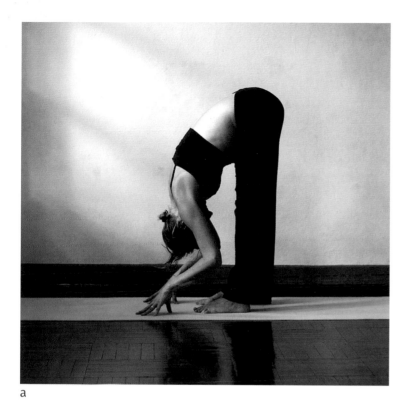

a

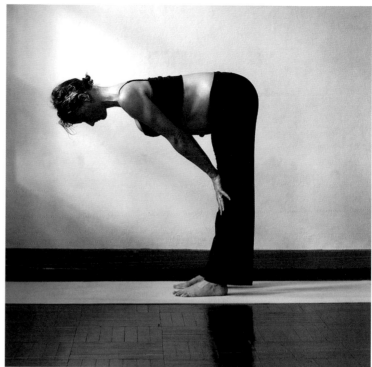

b

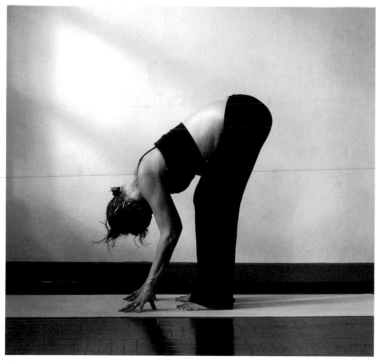

c

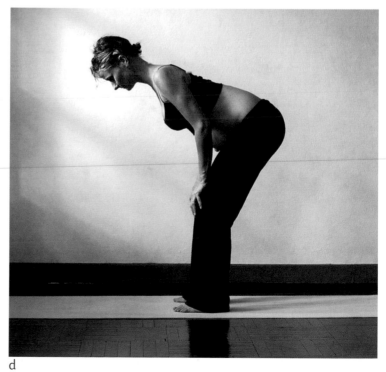

d

Reflection

*During our daily activities this week, we
explored moving our bodies through the pathways of
our spines.*

NAMASTÉ

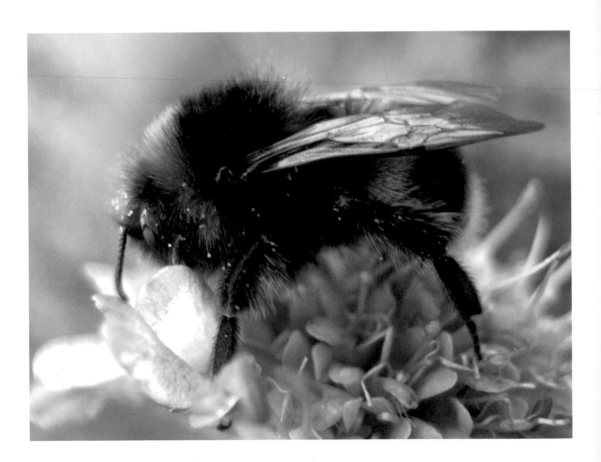

Grounding

*For the well-being of my growing baby, it is important for me to have
a balanced and healthy lifestyle.*

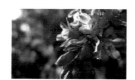

Playfully I will explore my hands and feet, spread my fingers and toes and share with you this practice centered on grounding.

As we journey together towards the end of the first trimester, I find comfort in knowing that the primary stages of your major organs are near to completion and you can concentrate on growing and getting stronger.

This week some of your vital organs begin to function independently.

The four love chambers of your heart are now formed, vigorously pumping blood through your body and your umbilical cord to the site where the placenta is growing, ready to connect you to me.

Your stomach is busy reorganizing itself, ready to attach to your mouth and intestines once they uncoil from your umbilical cord and re-enter your abdomen in a couple of weeks.

Like tiny buds your genitals begin to emerge this week. Although I won't know your sex until the next trimester, I am having fun guessing.

Your tiny fists uncurl, revealing little shoots of fingers. Like your toes they begin to separate and lose their webbed appearance, and you experience wriggling them for the very first time as you explore your hands and feet.

Although I won't be able to feel your movements for another month or so, I know that you are like a graceful acrobat, kicking and stretching in your bubble of fluid, playfully exploring your tiny limbs, fingers and toes.

Intention

This week, I will gently massage my feet with my hands
and invite my toes to separate between my fingers.
I will visualize tickling your tiny feet for the first time,
and wonder about all those magical journeys they will take you on.
I will imagine how our fingers will entwine around each other when they first meet,
and how with tactile tenderness your caressing little hands will explore the world.

Asana for the Week

Vrksasana – Tree Pose

BENEFITS: *Vrksasana opens the hips; strengthens the inner thighs and groin; calms the mind.*

CAUTIONS: *I will rest my raised foot against my ankle, calf or thigh, but not my knee. I will avoid this pose if I have pelvic girdle discomfort.*

MODIFICATIONS: *If I feel I may need some support to balance myself in this pose, I will use a chair or a wall to help me. These are useful props to use later on in my pregnancy, when my centre of gravity changes and I may find it is more difficult to balance.*

For this pose I will need a yoga mat and a chair or a wall to help steady myself.
    This pose is suitable for all stages of my pregnancy.

- ❁ Standing on my yoga mat, I check to make sure my feet are straight and parallel to each other.

- ❁ Looking at my toes, I lift them up, separate and spread them. Naturally I want to wriggle them, just as you are doing with your new toes.

- ❁ Playfully I explore bringing each one toe down individually.

- ❁ I ground down through my feet, connect with the earth and feel my foundation.

- ❁ I shift my weight over to the left, turn my right foot out and rest it on my left foot (a). Once I feel steady I begin to slide my right foot up the inside of my left leg and rest my right foot against my inner left thigh (b).

- ❁ Finding my balance I softly gaze at a focal point in front of me and bring my palms together in the gesture of Anjali mudra ('offering' or 'heart' mudra).

- ❁ Staying for five breaths, I mindfully repeat this week's affirmation:

For the well-being of my growing baby, it is important for me to have a
balanced and healthy lifestyle.

- ❁ I repeat the pose to the other side.

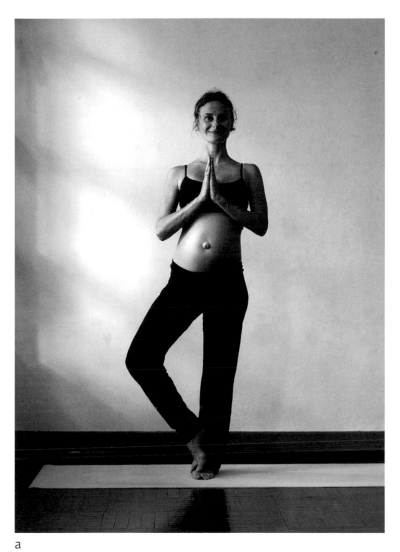

a

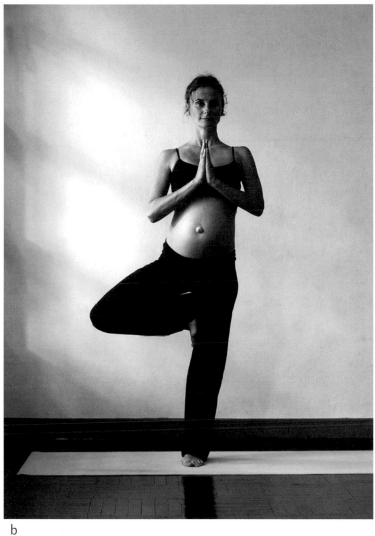

b

Reflection

This week my hands and feet were the foundation for my practice.
By spreading my fingers and toes I balanced, poised and connected with you as I
focused on grounding.

NAMASTÉ

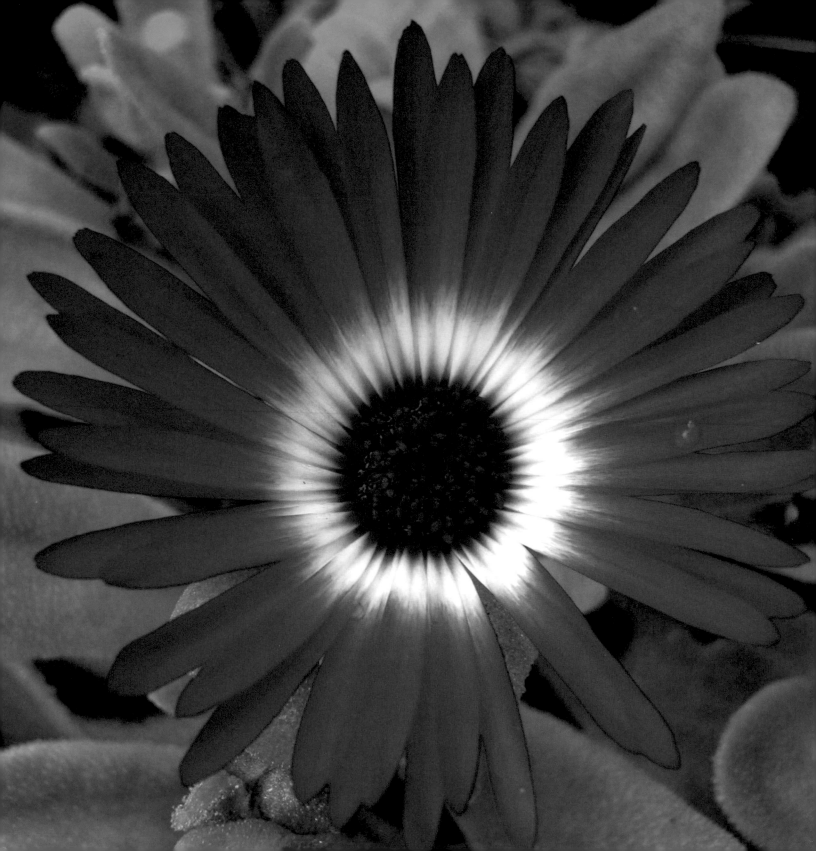

WEEK 12

The Pelvic Floor

When I smile my pelvic-floor muscles smile with me.

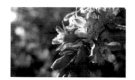

Forming a hammock-like structure at the base of my pelvic bowl is a network of muscles. These are instrumental to my health and my self-care as a woman – these are the muscles that form my pelvic floor.

Together we have reached the end of the first trimester. Slowly I am beginning to feel a little more like my familiar self again; the early symptoms of nausea and tiredness are gradually abating and I notice I have a little more energy.

Over the last few weeks you have been so busy creating your physical shape and internal organs that it is no wonder I have been so tired.

Your lifeline, your umbilical cord, is now attached to my small but complete placenta, connecting me to you, supplying you with all the essential hormones and nutrients you need to grow and taking away any harmful or unnecessary substances. This support system is essential to your well-being, and ensures that you have all you need to keep healthy and strong.

As you grow, so do I. My uterus is expanding to accommodate both you and my growing placenta. Now the size of a small grapefruit, my uterus is steadily changing shape and rising out of my pelvis. I am becoming aware of a slight swelling in my belly.

With the extra demands you will be placing on my pelvic organs and bladder over the following months, I remind myself of the importance of regularly practising the pelvic-floor exercises known as Kegel Exercises to help keep my pelvic-floor muscles healthy and active in readiness for your birth and my post-pregnancy care.

Intention

Today I will observe my daily habits:
putting the kettle on, brushing my teeth,
spending time with you;
 and I will choose one which will be my prompt
to perform my daily Kegel Exercises.

Practice for the Week

Kegel Exercises – Pelvic Floor Exercises

BENEFITS: *Kegel Exercises can increase the flexibility and elasticity of the pelvic-floor muscles, contributing to an easier birth and the prevention of tearing during delivery. Strengthening the muscles and learning to use them effectively can help to prevent instability of the pelvic floor during and after pregnancy. Practised post-birth, they can encourage the uterus to contract and return to its original shape, tone the abdomen and help with the healing process.*

For this pose I will need a yoga mat and several small cushions. I must remember to practise these exercises daily.

They are suitable for all stages of my pregnancy.

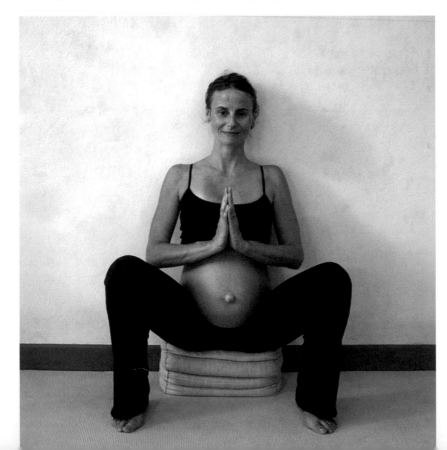

❀ Sitting with my back against a wall, I squat on several cushions and lovingly place my hands over you. I feel the tiny bump underneath that is you, and a smile rises up from inside of me.

❀ I bring my hands together in front of my heart in the Anjali mudra gesture. I take a moment to become familiar with my pelvic-floor muscles by imagining that I am peeing and wish to stop the flow of urine.

❀ I tense my jaw and notice my pelvic-floor muscles tightening, I smile and they release. I play a while at exploring the relationship between my facial muscles and those of my pelvic floor.

❀ Mindfully I repeat this week's affirmation:

When I smile my pelvic-floor muscles smile with me.

❀ I practise tightening and relaxing the muscles of my pelvic floor.

❀ I picture my pelvic floor as being divided into four levels and squeeze the muscles at each level, intensifying the squeeze as I move higher. At the top I pause, take a breath and slowly release back down through each level, squeezing for a count of five at each one. At the bottom I exhale fully, sending my breath down my body. I visualize my birth canal widening and expanding, creating a path for you to descend down.

❀ I feel my pelvic-floor muscles completely relax and I smile.

❀ On an inhalation I squeeze them so they contract, and on an exhalation I relax and release them. I repeat this for five breaths. Rapidly squeezing and releasing the muscles, I 'wink' with my pelvic floor for thirty counts. I hope to reach a hundred one day. These are my daily Kegel Exercises.

Reflection

*Through daily Kegel Exercises I am learning to:
strengthen, tone, relax, stimulate
and use effectively the muscles of
the pelvic floor.*

NAMASTÉ

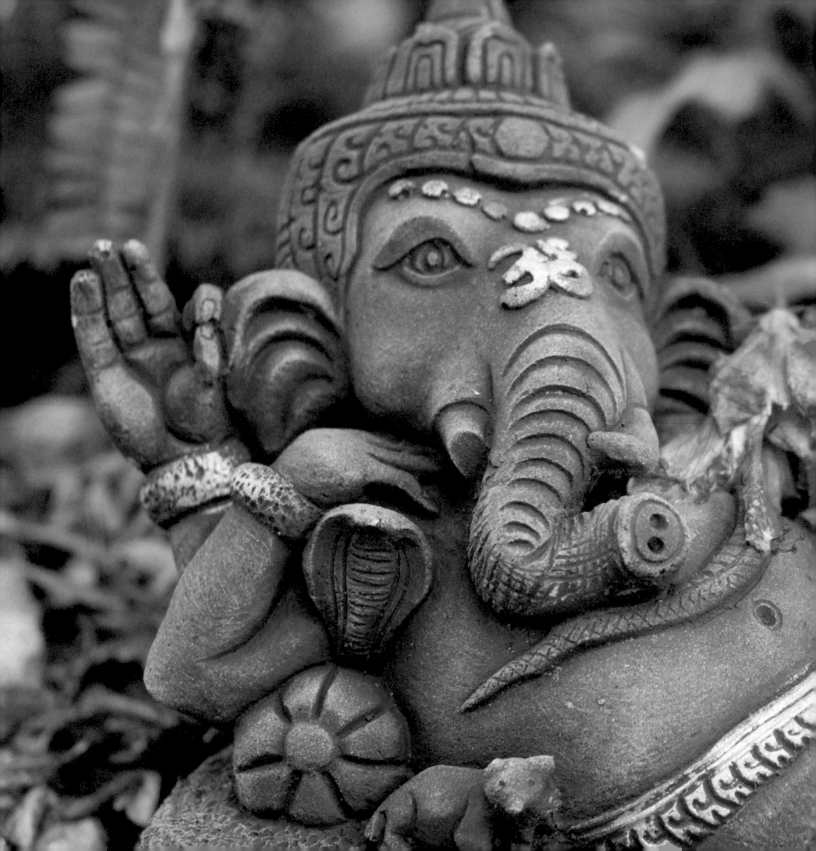

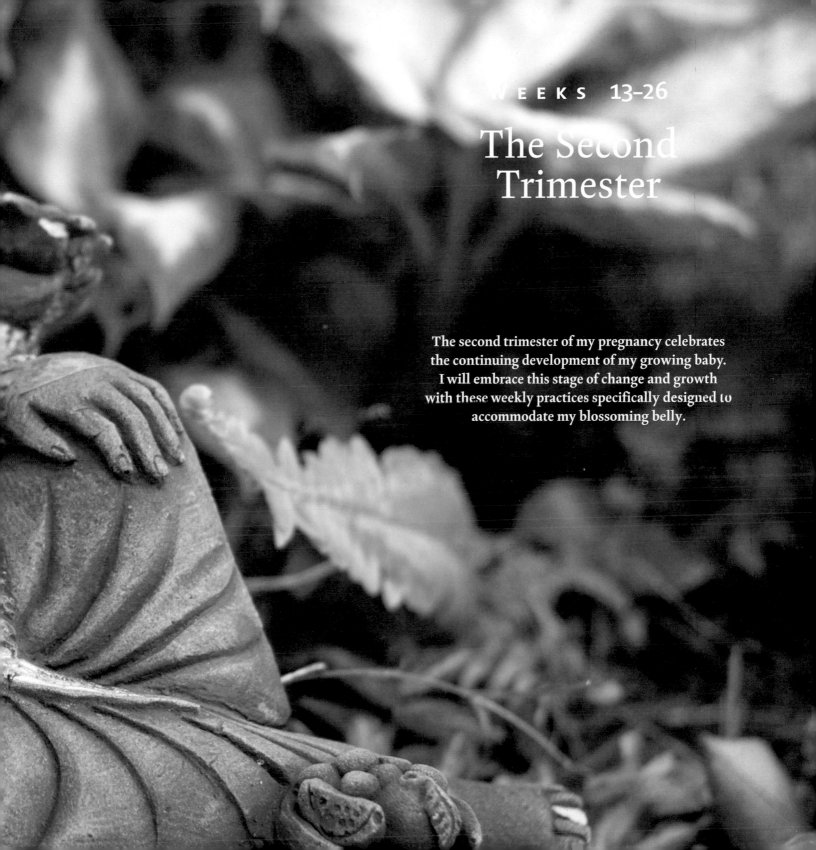

The Second Trimester

The second trimester of my pregnancy celebrates the continuing development of my growing baby. I will embrace this stage of change and growth with these weekly practices specifically designed to accommodate my blossoming belly.

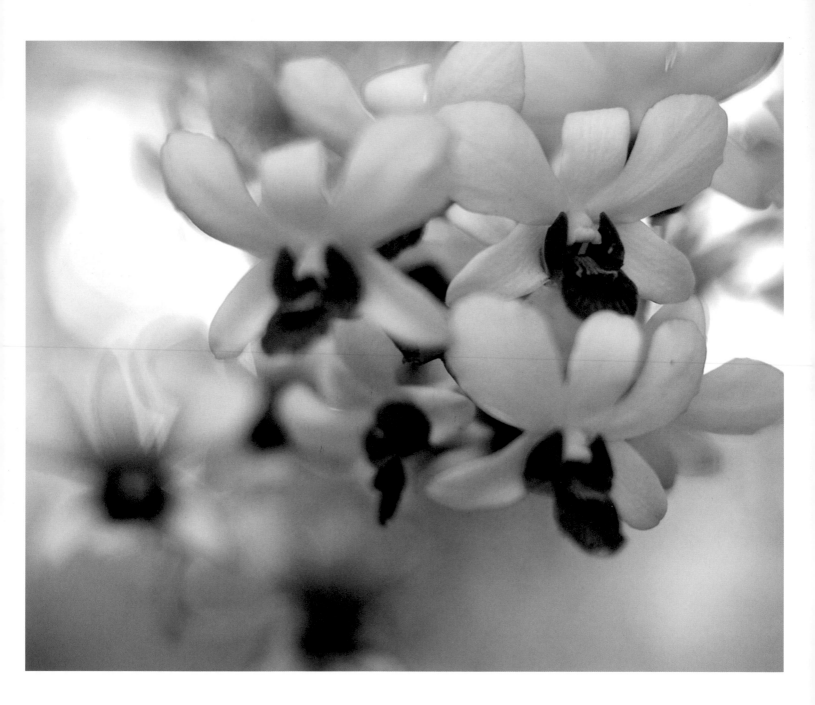

Our Digestive Systems

What is healthy for me is healthy for my growing baby.

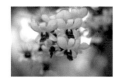

This week I will feed my soul with a practice that massages my internal organs and nourishes our digestive systems.

We are now in what is often called the honeymoon period of pregnancy.

As we embark on this new chapter of our journey together and my body gradually becomes accustomed to supporting you, I find myself wanting to relax a little, knowing that the foundations of your internal organs have been created. Diligently you focus on designing and sculpting their intricate characteristics and functions.

This week you concentrate on your digestive system.

Your intestines have now moved further into your body, finding their home and settling in your belly area. Although your digestive system is in place and links have been formed between your stomach, mouth and intestines, it will be a while before it all begins to function fully and for the time being you practise swallowing with small amounts of your amniotic fluid.

Your delicate little pancreas, the size of a small button, is busy producing insulin, the hormone needed to help you regulate your blood-sugar levels once you are born.

This reminds me that since my pancreas is currently supporting us both, I will work on curbing my sweet tooth and avoid excessive consumption of sugary foods.

While we are sharing the food I eat, I will be mindful of everything I consume, ensuring that my diet is balanced and full of rich nutrients and goodness to keep us both healthy and strong.

Intention

Together we will share a colourful plate of my favorite meal.
Mindfully I will chew each delicious mouthful,
savoring the richness of all the different flavors and textures.
In union our bodies will absorb all the nutritional goodness,
becoming replenished and refueled,
to help us grow healthier in our mind, body and spirit.

BENEFITS: *Prasarita Padottanasana stimulates the internal organs; tones the abdominal muscles; promotes a healthy digestive system; improves digestion and elimination; strengthens the spine; helps to relieve lower-back discomfort; stretches the inner and back leg muscles and lengthens the hamstrings.*

CAUTIONS: *If I have pelvic girdle discomfort I will take a narrower stance by bringing my feet outer-hip-width apart and I will use a block or seat of a chair to practise the pose (d).*

MODIFICATIONS: *If my spine rounds in this pose I will use blocks under my hands (c).*

Asana for the Week

Prasarita Padottanasana – Wide Angle Forward Bend with an Open Twist

For this pose I will need a yoga mat and two blocks.
This pose is suitable for all stages of my pregnancy.

❁ I take a wide stance along my yoga mat with my feet facing forward and parallel to each other.

❁ Tilting at my hips, I take a forward fold and rest my hands on the floor beneath my shoulders. I take a breath here (a).

❁ Keeping my hips level and belly soft, I keep my right hand on the floor and direct my upper chest over to the left as I open up into the twist.

❁ I raise my left arm up towards the sky and come into a full expression of the pose (b).

❁ On each inhalation I soften my belly and on each exhalation I let my internal organs and digestive system be gently massaged through the action of this open twist. I think of the network of your digestive system forming in your body.

❁ Staying for five breaths, I mindfully repeat this week's affirmation:

What is healthy for me is healthy for my growing baby.

❁ I repeat the open twist to my other side.

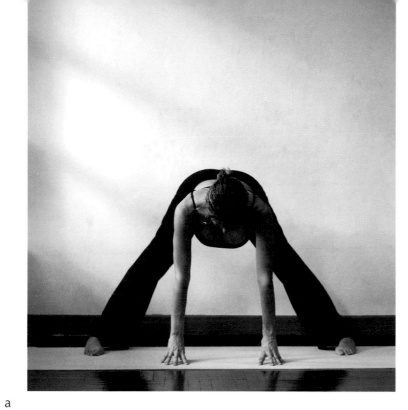

a

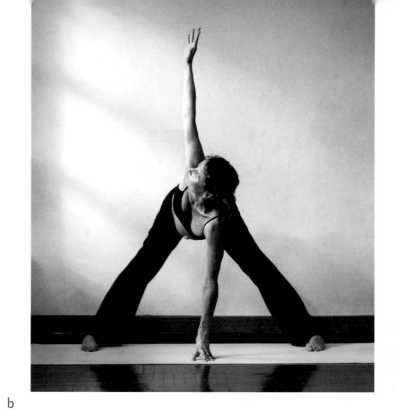

b

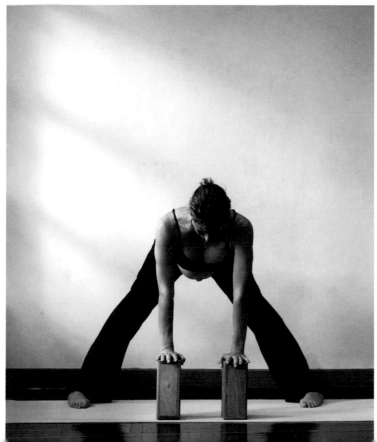

c

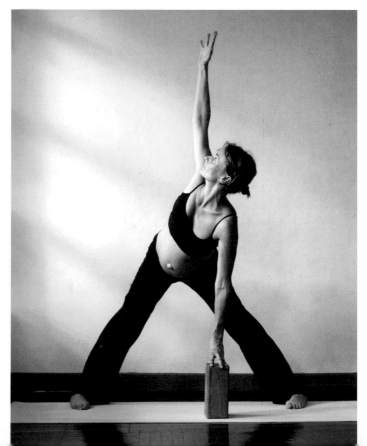

d

Reflection

Tasting the essence of my breath, I nourished my soul and enriched my being in a practice that honored our digestive systems.

NAMASTÉ

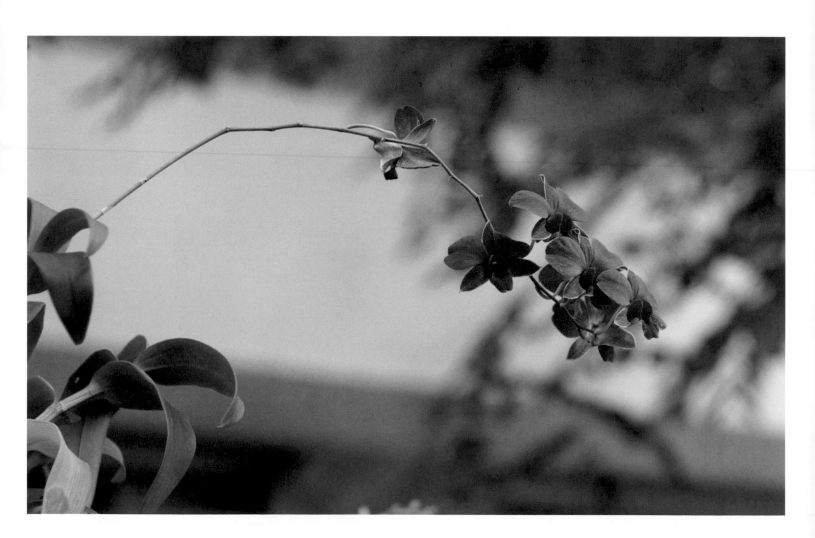

Our Faces

My body naturally relaxes when I smile.

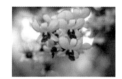

This week I will have fun, playfully exploring my facial expressions, uniting with you as we both practise exercising the muscles of our face.

Slowly I am adapting to all the different physical, emotional and spiritual changes that are taking place as my pregnancy progresses.

I am aware that my emotions reflect how I feel from the inside out and that I share all my thoughts and feelings with you. Each day I remind myself to stay calm and positive so you can be nurtured in a loving environment.

Up until now your head has always been a little larger than your body. Now, however, as your neck begins to lengthen and the shape of your head becomes more defined, they grow more in proportion to each other.

This week you channel your energy into developing the cast of your face.

Your sleeping eyes begin to journey forward towards the centre of your face – no need to open them yet though, there will be time for that later – and the sweet snub of your nose protrudes a little more, approaching its final maturity. You start to explore your new facial muscles with random and casual smiles, frowns and pouts.

Smiling, I think of you. I wonder what expression you are making now.

Intention

Each morning when I wash my face with cool water,
I will massage my facial features.
I will stand in front of a mirror
and make funny faces, I will smile, I will frown,
I will pout and I will blow a kiss to you.

BENEFITS: Laughing Yoga opens the chest; it relieves tension in the face, jaw and throat and stimulates the muscles of the face.

Asana for the Week

Laughing Yoga

For this pose I will need a yoga mat.

This pose is suitable for all stages of my pregnancy.

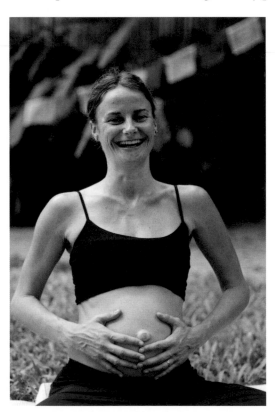

❀ I find a comfortable seat, place my hands lovingly around you and laugh.

❀ I begin with a little chuckle, which slowly grows into a hearty laugh.

❀ It is contagious; the more I laugh the more I want to laugh.

❀ Soon I find myself roaring with laughter and I feel my belly vibrate with my giggles.

❀ The muscles of my face are energized. I think of you exercising the muscles of your face as you laugh with me.

❀ I feel happy.

❀ Mindfully I repeat this week's affirmation:

My body naturally relaxes when I smile.

Reflection

Together we exercised our facial muscles and had fun expressing ourselves using our face.
NAMASTÉ

WEEK 15

Equanimity

My baby is growing in perfect proportion, becoming a healthy, whole and beautiful being.

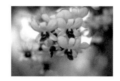

Our right side relates to the sun; our active, physical and masculine attributes. Our left side relates to the moon; our receptive, emotional and feminine qualities. By balancing and aligning them both I can enjoy equanimity.

Proportionally your skeleton is maturing.

Your muscles and bones are taking shape and your legs are lengthening and becoming longer than your arms.

You continue to refine the features of your face; the delicate structures of your ears begin to migrate to where they will be when you're born, and a shadow of faint fine hair forms your eyebrows.

Although your eyes will remain closed for several more months, you begin to sense light and dark, when day moves into night and the sun and moon cast shadows across my belly.

I am awash with hormones, either saturated with the female type or regulating the influx of male energy. My body adjusts to these changes as you begin to create your sexual organs.

If you are a girl, your very own uterus is now developing and your ovaries begin to move into your pelvic area. If you are a boy, a small swelling appears around now, signifying the beginnings of your genitals.

As I hold you in my hands I notice that my waistline is gradually disappearing as my belly changes shape, rounding a little more into a well-defined bump; a loving reminder that you are here with me.

Intention

This week I will be:
active and still,
serious and funny,
energetic and restful,
finding balance in my life,
in my work, rest and play.

Asana for the Week

Ardha Chandrasana – Half Moon Pose

For this pose I will need a yoga mat, a wall and a block or a chair to help steady myself. This pose is suitable for the first and second trimesters of my pregnancy.

❀ Placing my yoga mat against a wall, I take a wide stance with my feet facing forward and parallel to each other. I feel the support of the wall behind me.

❀ I turn my right foot out, aligning my front heel with the middle of the arch of my left foot.

❀ Wrapping my hands around you over my rounding belly, I check that both of my hips are facing into the center of the room.

❀ I take a breath.

❀ I ground down through my right foot, keeping my right leg straight.

❀ I steady myself, lean over to my right and place my right hand down on the floor a little way in front of my right little toe, so it is underneath my right shoulder.

❀ Finding my stability, I use the wall behind me for support and raise my left leg up to be level with my left hip.

❀ Holding you in my left hand I take a moment to find my balance.

❀ Slowly I raise my left arm up towards the sky and turn my upper chest up towards my left hand, finding my expression of the pose.

BENEFITS: Ardha Chandrasana strengthens the spine, ankles and thighs; opens the hips; stretches the groin, hamstrings, calves and shoulders; improves balance and calms the mind, helps to relieve pressure from the lower abdomen later in the second trimester.

MODIFICATIONS: If I am new to this pose, or in my second trimester, it is advised that I use the wall and a block or chair to support myself as demonstrated in (b) and (c).

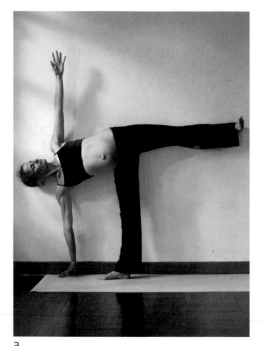
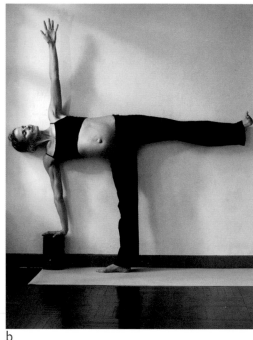
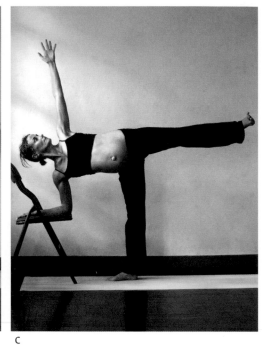

a

b

c

✽ Staying for five breaths, I mindfully repeat this week's affirmation:

My baby is growing in perfect proportion, becoming a healthy, whole and beautiful being.

✽ I repeat the pose to my other side.

Reflection

Through my practice of balance, I aligned my
right side with my left side to create an awareness of
wholeness, stability and equanimity.

NAMASTÉ

Our Circulation

*My circulation is flowing efficiently and effectively, continually sending
nourishment to my growing baby.*

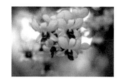

To complement the development of your internal systems, I will move my body with my breath in a rhythmical practice to help stimulate our circulation.

This month you will develop quickly, almost doubling your weight and growing longer in size.

Your skeletal structure is hardening, the cartilage changing from its original rubbery texture as it hardens into bone. Underneath your skin, layers of fat begin to accumulate, providing you with a perfect blanket of protection and insulation that keeps you warm and cozy.

As my circulatory system continues to support your growth, providing you with all the nutrients you need, your heart is working at pumping blood around your body.

By circulating the amniotic fluid and the oxygen you receive from me via your umbilical cord, your respiratory system is gradually strengthening, ready for when your lungs become fully mature later on in the third trimester.

While you practise breathing underwater you train yourself to swallow using the amniotic fluid. As you digest this, your urinary system rehearses the skill of filtering out unwanted items and you practise the process of urination.

While you continue to evolve, I notice my body changing too. My breasts are becoming fuller, filling with the precious fluid I will nurse you with, and as my uterus expands to make room for you, it puts a gentle squeeze on my bladder, making me want to empty it a little more often.

BENEFITS: The Cat Sequence strengthens and stretches the spine; helps relieve lower-back tension and helps alleviate pelvic girdle discomfort symptoms. It can be used in early labor to help alleviate back discomfort.

Intention

*This week I will go swimming
or take a long relaxing bath.
Bathing in the water,
I will think of you.
I will imagine you playing, moving and breathing,
floating in the buoyancy of your own oceanic world.*

Asana for the Week

Cat Sequence

For this pose I will need a yoga mat.

This pose is suitable for all stages of my pregnancy.

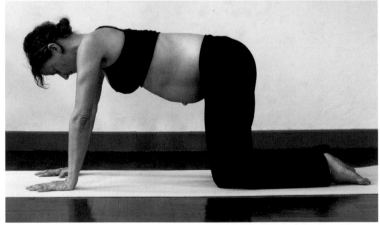

a

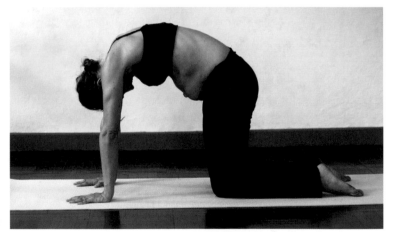

b

❁ I come onto all fours into a tabletop position.

❁ My hands are underneath my shoulders, the creases of my wrists are parallel to the front edges of my yoga mat and my knees are slightly wider than my hips (a).

❁ I inhale and direct my breath all the way down to you.

❁ Through my exhalation I scoop my tailbone under and round my spine, tucking my chin towards my chest and looking towards you (b).

❁ Letting my breath lead my body, I synchronize these movements with my breath. On my inhalations I return to (a), and with my exhalations I form the shape of (b).

❁ Rhythmically moving my body through this sequence five times, mindfully I repeat this week's affirmation:

My circulation is flowing efficiently and effectively, continually sending nourishment to my growing baby.

Reflection

This week I synchronized moving my body with the rhythm of my breath to encourage the flow of our circulation.

NAMASTÉ

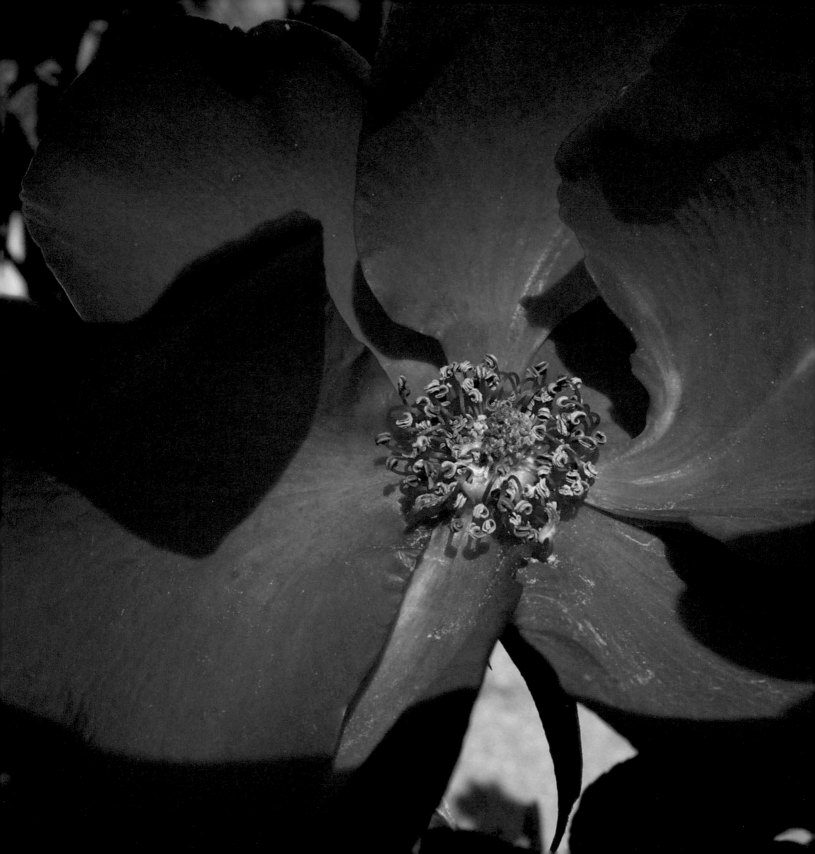

Our Nervous Systems

*Each sensation I feel of my growing baby moving reassures me
that all is well.*

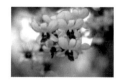

By slowing down, resting and restoring my mind, body and soul a message of relaxation will be conveyed to our nervous systems.

Behind my growing belly your physical make-up is steadily maturing.

Your focus this week is your nervous system, with the development of a protective white covering – myelin – which begins to cloak your nerve cells.

This covering means that more connections between your mind and body are ignited and faster messages can be sent. You learn to respond to both internal and external cues as your primary impulses begin to evolve.

Involuntarily you learn to yawn, and underneath your closed eyelids your eyes begin to flicker with the discovery of the blinking reflex.

Each day you are becoming more limber, and move with more intention.

Like a little yogi you are making pretzel shapes with your body; twisting, stretching, folding and reaching while you discover and play with your first toy – the umbilical cord.

I may soon start to feel you moving inside me. I eagerly wait for this moment and find quiet times in my busy life to pause. Resting my hands over my belly I wait. For a fleeting minute I feel you moving inside me, a quickening sensation, like a succession of tiny air bubbles tiptoeing inside my belly.

BENEFITS: *Viparita Karani regulates blood flow; improves circulation; relaxes the nervous system; calms the mind; helps alleviate swollen ankles and calves; rests tired legs.*

CAUTIONS: *It is advised that I do not practise this pose after week 34 of my pregnancy or once my baby is engaged.*

Intention

I take a rest and place my hands over my belly.
I tell you how much I love you.
I wait for your response:
a gentle kick; a hiccup; a tender prod.
Thank you, I love you.

Asana for the Week

Viparita Karani – The Great Rejuvenator

For this pose I will need a yoga mat, a wall, several small cushions and an eye pillow.
   This pose is suitable for all stages of my pregnancy.

❀ I sit sideways beside a wall with my legs extended out in front of me and right hip and shoulder against the wall. Pivoting at my hips, I swing my legs up the wall and lie down. I lift my hips and place several cushions under my pelvis. I place a folded blanket under my head and let my arms rest alongside my body.

❀ I place an eye pillow over my closed eyes.

❀ Resting my hands over you, I sense you beneath my touch.

❀ I practise this week's intention, telling you how much I love you, and listen for your response.

❀ Staying here for up to fifteen minutes, I mindfully repeat this week's affirmation:

   Each sensation I feel of my growing baby moving reassures me that all is well.

❀ To come out of the pose, I bend my knees and rest my feet against the wall. I lift my hips, remove the cushions from under my pelvis, then roll over to my left side. I stay here for a few minutes before using my hands to gently assist me up into a sitting position.

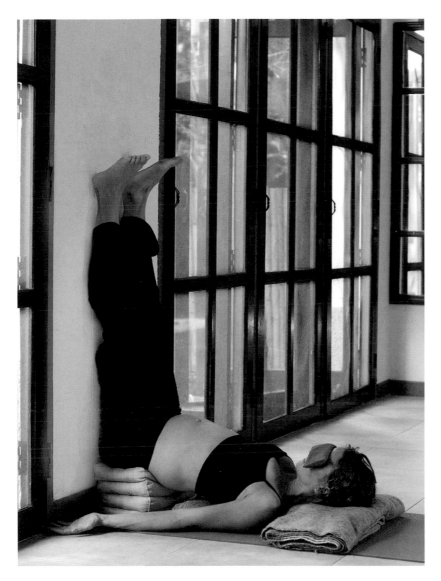

Reflection

This week I relaxed and re-energized
with a restorative practice, which calmed and recharged
our nervous systems.

NAMASTÉ

WEEK 18

The Vibration of Sound

My baby is listening when I say, "I love you".

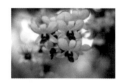

Letting go of my inhibitions, I will let my soul sing and let my growing baby be soothed with my voice through the vibration of sound.

Your ears are now sitting proudly at the side of your head. The bones of your inner ear and their nerve endings have formed and you are becoming sensitive to sound. A particular area in your brain has been allocated to enable you to tune in to the noises of your world.

The sound of my heart beating, my blood circulating, my stomach churning and the muffled murmurings of my voice – all of these are becoming familiar comforters to you.

I play some relaxing, calming music to you while you are in the womb; maybe it will be a soothing lullaby for you once you are born.

Each week you are growing stronger. Your bones are hardening with calcium deposits as the process of ossification continues, and your muscles strengthen and lengthen from your repetitive and vigorous movements.

As my pregnancy progresses it is important that I continue to be sensitive to both our needs, listen to the wisdom of my body and respect the physical changes taking place.

I no longer rest flat on my back; this helps to keep our circulation flowing freely.

Instead I rest on my left side, my moon side, the side that connects me to my heart. Wrapping my arms around you, we soon drift off to sleep as I chant the mantra, "I love you".

Intention

I will play to you my favorite music.
I will sing to you a soothing lullaby.
I will chant the mantra, "I love you",
and together we will gently sway to the rhythm of our hearts.

Pranayama for the Week

The Birthing Breath

For this pose I will need a yoga mat, a wall and several small cushions.
   This breathing exercise is suitable for all stages of my pregnancy.

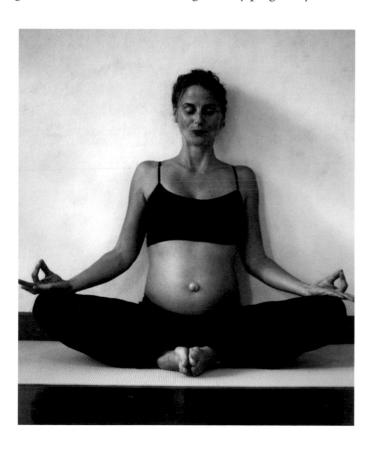

BENEFITS: *The Birthing Breath soothes the nervous system; focuses and calms the mind; improves concentration and helps to balance emotions.*
It is a useful breathing technique to use in labor.
Using deep vowel sounds, as in this practice, can be a valuable tool during labor to help direct the energy down to the base of the body and help to relax the pelvic-floor muscles to ease delivery.

CAUTIONS: *If I have pelvic girdle discomfort I will practise this breathing exercise sitting on my heels with my knees together. I will place a cushion(s) between my sitting bones and my heels to bridge any gaps.*

❀ Sitting with my back against a wall, I bring the soles of my feet together.

❀ I rest the backs of my hands on my thighs, and bringing the tip of each thumb to touch the tip of my index finger I extend my other three fingers. This hand gesture is known as Jnana mudra, and symbolizes the uniting of our unconscious with our conscious energy.

❀ I close my eyes and connect with my breath. Parting my lips and teeth slightly, I soften my mouth. Inhaling naturally through my nose, I exhale through my mouth, directing the sensation of the exhalation down past you to my pelvic floor.

❀ I visualize and sense my pelvic floor softening and releasing with each exhalation.

❀ I let my inhalations come in naturally through my nose and focus on exhaling through my mouth.

❀ I notice that my exhalations are longer when I breathe out through my mouth, and that this makes me feel more relaxed.

❀ I repeat this breath five times.

❀ Letting go of my inhibitions, I begin to sound the vowel "ooo" along with my exhalation and feel it vibrate through my body down to my pelvic floor. How does it sound to you? I repeat this five times, then I repeat it making the sound "aaahhh" five times.

❀ I find each sound soothing and calming.

❀ Mindfully I repeat this week's affirmation:

My baby is listening when I say, "I love you".

❀ Gradually my breath settles back into its natural rhythm.

Reflection

This week my voice reverberated through my practice and connected with my growing baby with the vibration of sound.

NAMASTÉ

WEEK 19

Our Senses

I am sensitive to my needs and the needs of my growing baby.

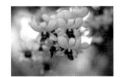

Through seeing, hearing, tasting and feeling we will unite in a practice that stimulates our senses.

Over the last couple of weeks you have enjoyed the wonders of your maturing nervous system. A flowing traffic of messages is being constantly exchanged between your mind and body as countless more nerves come into existence. This week you have five new gifts to play with: your senses. Your brain is choosing a place for each single one. Over time you will become increasingly sensitive and responsive to external sounds, light, touch, smells and the taste from my food.

Concentrating on growing stronger, you have more of an appetite and are keen to absorb the goodness of the food we share.

You have acquired quite a taste for the amniotic fluid from swallowing, digesting and excreting it. Sometimes you drink it a little too quickly and give yourself hiccups, which I recognize from the rhythmical pulsations quickening across my tummy.

As you become bigger so does my uterus, which is about the size of a honeydew melon now. Occasionally I experience a twinge like stitch around my lower belly, as the ligaments supporting my uterus stretch to make a little more room for you.

To help with this my body releases the hormone relaxin, which naturally loosens my ligaments and other connective tissue. My body is naturally becoming more flexible, preparing to be open and ready for you, so I must be careful not to overstretch in my yoga practice.

BENEFITS: *Adho Mukha Svanasana stretches the shoulders, front and back leg muscles; lengthens the spine; strengthens the arms and legs; helps relieve lower-back tension; calms the mind and rejuvenates the body.*

MODIFICATIONS: *If my spine rounds in this pose or I feel an intense stretch down the back of my legs, I will bend my knees and lift my heels up (b).*

Intention

Together we will take a gentle walk and awaken our senses.
With each fragrance I smell your nose may twitch,
with each image I see your eyes may blink,
with each sound I hear your ears may listen,
with each breath I take our hearts will beat,
with each step I take I sense you moving beneath my skin
and with each sentiment I feel my love for you will deepen.

Asana for the Week

Adho Mukha Svanasana – Downward Facing Dog

For this pose I will need a yoga mat.

This pose is suitable for the first and second trimesters of my pregnancy.

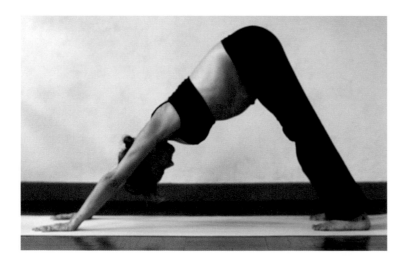

a

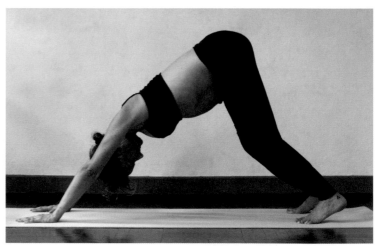

b

✿ I come onto all fours into a tabletop position; my hands are underneath my shoulders and my knees slightly wider than my hips.

✿ I position my knees behind my hips.

✿ I check to ensure that the creases of my wrists are parallel with the front edge of my yoga mat. Spreading my fingers, I ground down through my fingertips and base knuckles and feel the texture of the floor beneath my hands.

✿ I turn my toes under and lift my hips up towards the sky, coming into an inverted v-shape.

✿ I lengthen my spine and straighten my legs, feeling the stretch along the back of my legs.

✿ I ground through the ball of my big toe and little toe with the intention of drawing my heels down towards the earth, and feel the texture of the floor beneath my feet.

✿ In this shape I am upside down and I wonder if you are too.

✿ I feel a sense of lightness in my belly. How does it feel for you?

✿ Staying for five breaths, I mindfully repeat this week's affirmation:

I am sensitive to my needs and the needs of my growing baby.

Reflection

*This week I was sensitive to my world around me
and the world of you inside me,
uniting with you in a practice through all of
our senses.*

NAMASTÉ

WEEK 20

A Loving Touch

The complex nature of my growing baby's skin is perfecting itself for my loving touch.

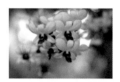

To signify the creation of the more delicate features of the fingers and toes, I will bring my hands together into a gesture of a loving touch.

We are now halfway through your wonderful journey of creation.

This week I shall take a peek into your world again with another pregnancy ultrasound scan. I shall see how you have grown; the delicate features of your face, your dainty fingers and toes. I may even be able to confirm the secret of your sex – if I choose to ask.

I am so proud of all you have achieved over the last few months; growing from a tiny cell into my baby. Many of your internal organs are physically complete and they are functioning independently, so now you can begin to concentrate on their more intricate features.

Your body is coated in a waxy layer called vernix caseosa, and a layer of delicate, fine fluffy hairs known as lanugo adorns your body. Both of these help to protect your delicate skin and keep you warm.

Ridges appear on your fingers and toes where your nails will be, and you make padding on your hands and feet.

Incidentally, I notice that my own nails are growing stronger and my hair appears thicker, fuller and healthier thanks to all those pregnancy hormones, which add nutrients and nourishment to my cells too.

Intention

Treating myself to a manicure this week,
I will marvel at the ridges on my fingers and lines on my hands,
which they say reveal a tale of my life.
I wonder what life story your hands will hold.

Asana for the Week

Malasana – Squat or Garland Pose

For this pose I will need a yoga mat, a blanket and a wall.

✾ I take a squat position. My feet are wider than my hips and I turn them out to ensure that you have enough room to be comfortable.

BENEFITS: *Malasana stretches the groin, inner thighs and hips and strengthens the thighs.*

CAUTIONS: *I will avoid this pose if I have any knees injuries or pelvic girdle discomfort. It is advised I do not practise deep or unsupported squats after week 34 of my pregnancy or once my baby is engaged.*

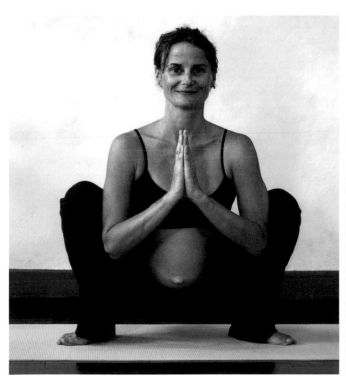

a

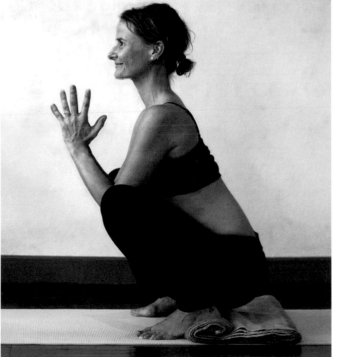

b

❀ I check to make sure my knees are pointing over my second and third toes and my spine is straight.

❀ If my heels do not rest on the floor when I squat, I will roll up a blanket and place it to bridge the gaps between the floor and my heels (b).

❀ I stroke my belly and think of you. I notice the tenderness of my touch as I feel the softness and smoothness of my hands lovingly caressing you.

❀ Bringing my hands together in front of my heart center in a gesture of a loving touch known as Anjali mudra (a), I feel my right hand lovingly touch my left hand, and my left lovingly touch my right hand as I marry the two together.

❀ Staying for five breaths, I mindfully repeat this week's affirmation:

The complex nature of my growing baby's skin
is perfecting itself for my loving touch.

Reflection

This week I became sensitive to the sensations in the soles of my feet
and the palms of my hands, uniting with you through an act of
a loving touch. NAMASTÉ

Resounding Strength

My baby is growing stronger every day.

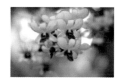

The resilience of my body to support my growing baby will be expressed in this practice, which is fuelled by power, passion and resounding strength.

This stage of my pregnancy is lovely; my body has adjusted to being pregnant, the general discomforts from the first trimester have gone and I am feeling more comfortable with my new body image.

With each day I am growing more in tune with your gentle kicks, all of them loving reminders of how beautiful you are, unfolding and growing inside of me. A trail of my voice echoes inside your home, like soft murmurings, a sound you are now very familiar with.

Your slight pink mouth has taken shape, with a double curve known as Cupid's bow forming on your upper lip. I will adore this each time I kiss you. Your eyebrows and eyelids are complete. For the time being, though, you will keep your eyes softly closed, gently opening them in time for your birth-day when our gazes will meet.

Since all your limbs have now developed, at our monthly check-ups from now on your growth will be measured from head to heel, rather than crown to rump.

You are forever in my thoughts and I send messages to you, reassuring you that all is well and telling you how much you are loved as our relationship of mother and child strengthens.

How blessed I am to carry you around so close to my heart for these nine months.

BENEFITS: *Virabhadrasana I stretches the hamstrings, hips and calves; strengthens the thighs and lengthens the spine.*

CAUTIONS: *After week 34 I will practise this pose by straddling a chair with my right sitting bone and the top of my right thigh resting on the seat of the chair, then repeating the pose to my other side.*
I will avoid this pose if I have pelvic girdle discomfort.

MODIFICATIONS: *To help steady myself in this pose I can rest my back heel against a wall and look forward.*
If I have high blood pressure it is advised that I practise this pose with my hands on my hips.

Intention

Like a warrior
I am triumphant and strong.
Protecting and shielding you
with the armor of my body,
as you continue to grow healthy and strong.

Asana for the Week

Virabhadrasana I – Warrior 1

For this pose I will need a yoga mat and a chair or a wall.

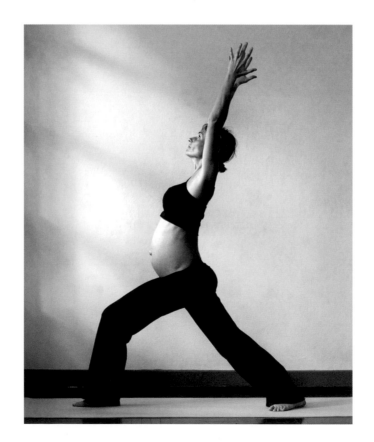

- Standing at the top of my yoga mat, I step my left foot back and turn it out at a slight angle.
- I check that both of my hips are facing forward.
- I place my hands around you and feel my expanding belly.
- I take a breath, honoring my body's flexibility, strength and resilience and its ability to carry, support and protect you.
- Inhaling, I draw upon these qualities.
- Exhaling, I bend my right knee, ensuring that it is stacked directly above my right ankle and aligned with my second and third toes.
- Grounding down through my right foot and through the outside edge of my left foot, I find my stability. I raise my arms above my head.
- I feel strength from my waist down towards the earth, and at the same time a sense of lightness up from my waist and through my fingertips. I look up towards my hands.
- Staying for five breaths, I mindfully repeat this week's affirmation:

  My baby is growing stronger every day.

- I repeat the pose to my other side.

Reflection

In a practice infused with energy, vigor and enthusiasm
I celebrated the ability of my body
to continually support you with
resounding strength.

NAMASTÉ

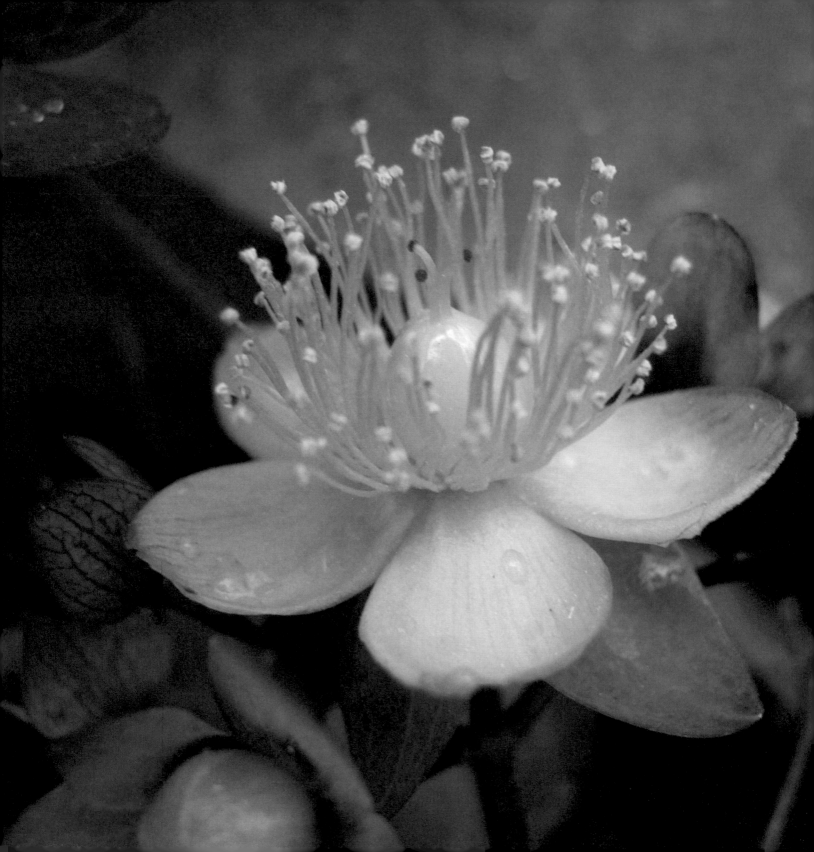

Feeling Radiant

I am a beautiful pregnant woman.

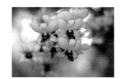

As a woman I carry compassion, kindness, power and beauty within me. In my practice this week I will reaffirm these qualities and enjoy feeling radiant.

Even though your organs are now formed and functioning, your brain is still developing.

Your sense of touch is perfecting itself and you have fun feeling and exploring the texture of your skin, body parts and your favorite toy, the umbilical cord.

Tastebuds have appeared on your tongue and your baby teeth are like hidden jewels beneath your gums.

As you grow, my little one, so do I. My uterus is stretching and feels uncomfortable and itchy – I use natural aloe vera to help alleviate this – and even my belly button is popping out now. Not to worry though, I've been told that it is likely to revert to being an inny after your birth-day.

I do feel radiant though. My cheeks feel flushed, my face is beaming, my hair gleaming – together we are blossoming!

BENEFITS: *Utkata Konasana strengthens the spine, ankles, thighs and shoulders; opens the hips; stretches the groin, inner thighs and opens the chest.*

CAUTIONS: *If I have pelvic girdle discomfort I will take a narrower stance by bringing my feet outer-hip-width apart.*
It is advised that I do not practise deep or unsupported squats after week 34 of my pregnancy or once my baby is engaged.

MODIFICATIONS: *If I am new to this pose or in my third trimester, it is advised that I rest my back against a wall to help steady myself (b).*
If I have high blood pressure it is advised that I practise this pose with my hands on my hips.

Intention

Sitting quietly I will bring my hands together in front of my heart.
Closing my eyes I will look within myself
and feel my heart beat from the inside.
I will visualize the golden glow shining from my heart
beaming out in all directions, in all dimensions.
I will share this light generously with everyone I meet this week,
and I will share it with you.
Always.

Asana for the Week

Utkata Konasana – Goddess Pose

For this pose I will need a yoga mat and a wall.

❀ Taking a wide stance along my yoga mat with my feet facing forward and parallel to each other, I turn my feet out at a slight angle, making sure that the heels are in line with each other.

❀ I bend my knees, stacking them directly above my ankles and ensuring that they are aligned with my second and third toes.

❀ I bend my elbows and bring them in line with my shoulders. I point my fingers up towards the sky with my palms facing forward and come into the full expression of the pose (a).

❀ I feel the blossoming of my belly and the radiance of carrying you inside me shining out through my entire being.

❀ Staying for five breaths, I mindfully repeat this week's affirmation:

I am a beautiful pregnant woman.

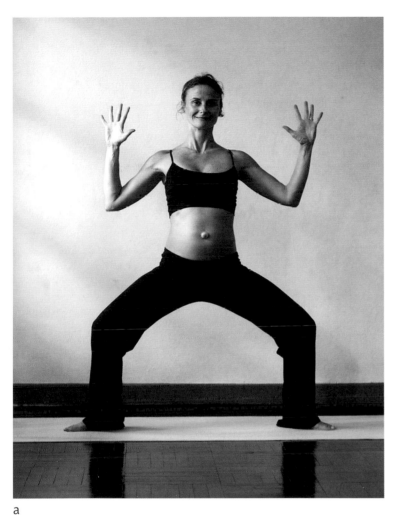

a

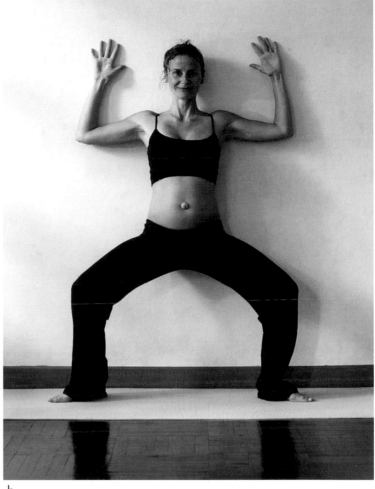

b

Reflection

Glowing from the blooming stage of my pregnancy
I expressed my inner and outer beauty in this practice, which left me
feeling radiant.

NAMASTÉ

Return to Center

I accept all of my unwelcomed emotions as a reminder to stay positive and confident in my ability to have the birth I desire.

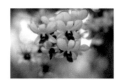

Sometimes I may find myself feeling a little off-center in my pregnancy both physically and emotionally, so this week I will find ways to realign my feelings to help me return to center.

Even though you still have a lot of growing and development to do and you could fit into the palm of my hand, your body now resembles that of a newborn.

Your digestive system continues to mature, absorbing valuable nutrients from me, and your tiny pancreas is now fully functioning, controlling your sugar levels. To help us both maintain a healthy, balanced diet, I am resisting the urge for sweet snacks and eating healthy alternatives instead.

Your skin is still translucent and quite red in appearance. Although for now it is heavily wrinkled and too big, you will begin to fill out and iron out the wrinkles in your skin over the next couple of weeks, when you start to deposit layers of fat and put on weight. I am sure my skin would be wrinkled too, if I had been swimming for the last twenty-three weeks!

The bones of your inner ear are hardening as your hearing becomes more refined and your sense of balance develops. Did you know that the bones in your inner ear become the hardest bones in your body?

As you and I grow, my center of gravity shifts both physically and emotionally. Sometimes I find myself feeling a little off balance, weeping unexpectedly at the smallest thing. I try to adjust to these ongoing changes by reminding myself to stay centered physically, emotionally and spiritually, and simply allowing any unwelcome feelings to pass by.

Intention

This week I shall slow down from the momentum of my life.
I will take time to come back to my center,
to prepare my mind, body and soul
for the next big adventure in my life;
motherhood.

Asana for the Week

Parivrtta Sukhasana – Revolved Easy Twist

For this pose I will need a yoga mat and a small cushion(s).

This pose is suitable for all stages of my pregnancy.

BENEFITS: *Parivrtta Sukhasana improves digestion and elimination; lengthens the spine, helps relieve lower-back tension; calms the mind and helps balance emotions.*

CAUTIONS: *If I have pelvic girdle discomfort I will practise this pose sitting on my heels with my knees together. I will place a cushion(s) between my sitting bones and my heels to bridge any gaps.*

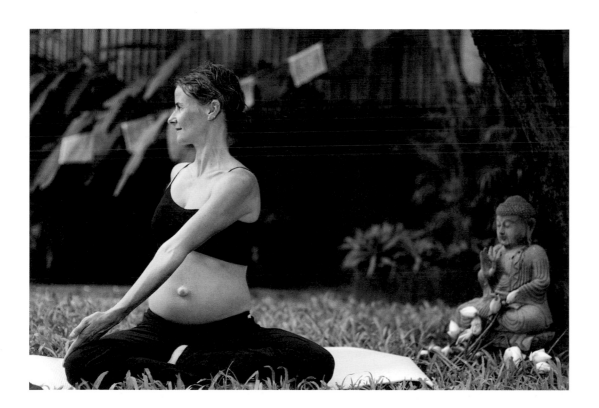

❀ Sitting in a comfortable cross-legged position, I bring my hands to my belly; to you. I observe how I am feeling physically, emotionally and mentally.

❀ Scanning my body with my mind, I notice any areas of tension and become a 'witness' to my thoughts, observing them without judging.

❀ I connect with my breath; with each inhalation I fill my body with love, compassion and kindness and with each exhalation I invite softness into my body and let go of any unwanted thoughts or emotions.

❀ Inhaling, I root down through my sitting bones and lengthen my spine.

❀ Exhaling, I turn my upper chest to the right.

❀ I bring my left hand to rest on my right knee and my right hand to rest behind my left sitting bone.

❀ My gaze follows me as I turn.

❀ Staying for five breaths, I mindfully repeat this week's affirmation:

> *I accept all of my unwelcome emotions as a reminder to stay positive and confident in my ability to have the birth I desire.*

❀ When I come out of the twist I enjoy the sensation of feeling centered and aligned. I remind myself that whatever feels twisted, distorted or out of sorts in my life can also be untwisted.

❀ I repeat the pose to my other side.

Reflection

Through my practice I was able to ground myself, connect to my core and find stability to help me return to center.

NAMASTÉ

WEEK 24

Creating Space

My body naturally makes room for my growing baby.

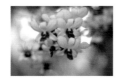

As my body accommodates the growth of my baby and I begin to make room in my life to be your mother, I will dedicate my practice to creating space.

This week the respiratory trees of your lungs, the alveoli, start to branch out and grow, forming air sacs and a network of blood vessels to help you breathe later on. For the time being you rehearse breathing with a special fluid made by your lungs, your delicate little chest gently rising and falling with the action.

As you practise the mechanism of breathing, I on the other hand notice how I sometimes find myself becoming out of breath as I go about my daily tasks, my lungs and internal organs naturally becoming squashed as my body makes extra room for you to grow.

Looking at my bump I like to imagine unzipping my belly, down my linea nigra, a dark decorative streak that runs from belly button to pubic area, to take a peep inside your world. I dream about what you may look like and all that you are experiencing; the sound of my rushing blood, the gurgling of my digestive system, my heart pumping and the tenderness of my warm touch.

When I instinctively tune in to your times of playfulness and rest, I enjoy my own stillness as I stop what I'm doing and treasure these moments of our togetherness.

BENEFITS: *Trikonasana strengthens the spine; opens the hips; stretches the inner thighs, groin, hamstrings, calves and shoulders.*

CAUTIONS: *I will avoid this pose if I have pelvic girdle discomfort. If I have high blood pressure it is advised that I practise the pose with my on hands on my hips.*

MODIFICATIONS: *If I am new to this pose or would like help to steady myself in it, it is advised that I use a block or a chair for support (b) or (c).*

Intention

Preparing my nest for you to rest in,
I create space in my home for you and all that you will be.
I will extend my life to be your mother
and I open my heart to you.

Asana for the Week

Trikonasana – Triangle Pose

For this pose I will need a yoga mat and a block or a chair.
   This pose is suitable for all stages of my pregnancy.

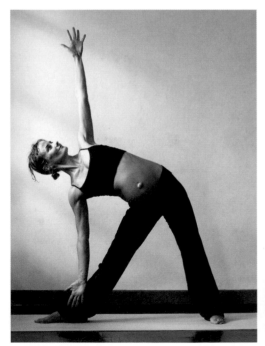

a

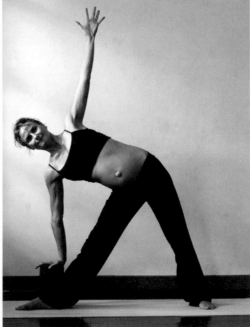

b

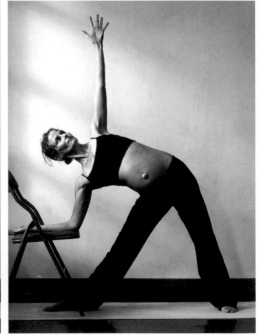

c

✽ I take a wide stance along my yoga mat with my feet facing forward and parallel to each other.

✽ I turn my right foot out, aligning my front heel with the middle of the arch of my left foot.

✽ I hold you in my hands and check both of my hips are facing into the center of the room.

✽ I lean over towards my right, letting my right arm slide down my right leg until it comes to rest along my right shin.

✽ I breathe into my belly, directing my breath down to you.

✽ On my inhalation I feel the fullness of my breath filling my belly.

✽ I sense it creating space inside my body for you.

✽ On my exhalation I soften into the pose.

✽ Slowly I lift my left arm up and come into my expression of the pose (a).

✽ Staying for five breaths, I mindfully repeat this week's affirmation:

My body naturally makes room for my growing baby.

✽ I repeat the pose to my other side.

Reflection

By finding freedom in my body and fullness in my breath,
I became open to the practice of
creating space.

NAMASTÉ

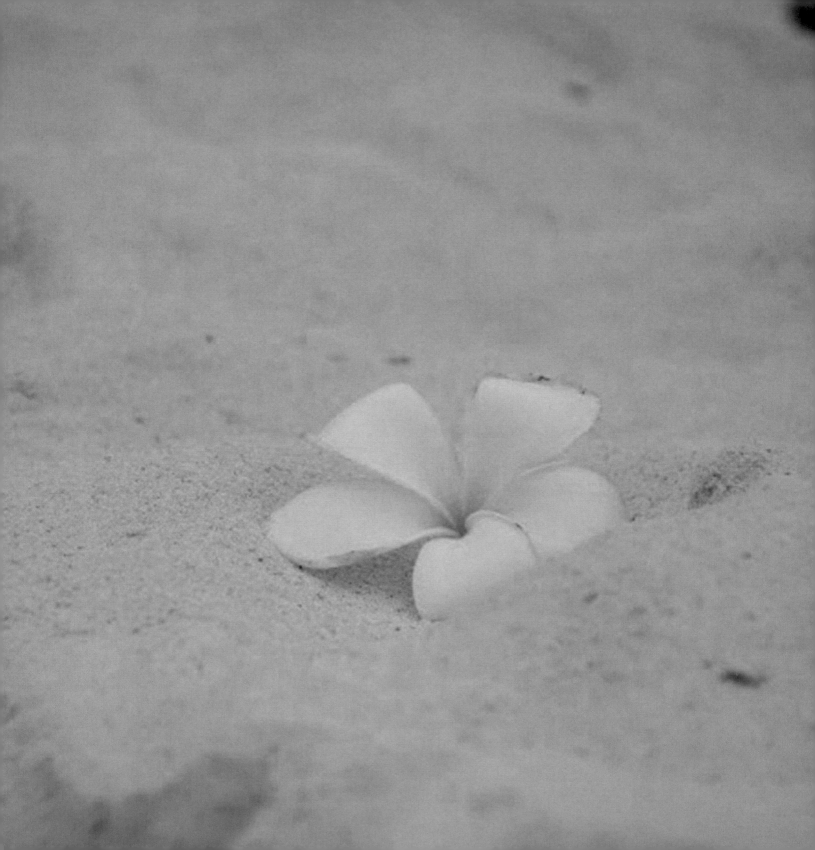

The Pelvis

My pelvis is designed to fit the shape of my baby's head.

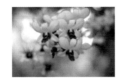

This week I will move freely from the point where my upper and lower body meet, where movement in the spine is initiated and where my precious growing baby is cradled in the pelvis.

Your spine is becoming more sophisticated; billions of nerves continue to form pathways from your organs to your brain and vice versa, and as a result your movements are becoming more controlled and coordinated and you are increasingly sensitive to touch, sound and taste.

To refine your movements you repeatedly practise stretching, reaching and kicking.

Often I like to spend time talking to you and stroking my belly waiting for you to answer, so we can play a while together.

My uterus is the size of a volleyball now, which can put extra strain on my lower back and pressure on my pelvis. My pelvis is supporting the weight of us both and is the entrance to the birth journey you will undertake.

It is important, therefore, that I am mindful of maintaining good posture, both during my everyday activities and when I exercise, so that I do not overstretch my pelvic area. I also continue with my daily Kegel Exercises (see pages 40/41).

I will remember to lie on my left side during rest and support myself with cushions under my belly and between my legs. I will also be careful not to do any unnecessary lifting, twisting or bending.

BENEFITS: *Standing Pelvic Rotations help relieve lower-back tension; improve mobility in the pelvis; release the hips and the pelvic girdle.*

Intention

Letting go of my inhibitions,
I will move like a belly dancer;
circulating my hips, rotating my pelvis
and moving my body to its own exquisite rhythm.

Asana for the Week

Standing Pelvic Rotations

For this pose I will need a yoga mat.

This pose is suitable for all stages of my pregnancy.

❀ Standing on my yoga mat with my feet slightly wider than hip distance apart, I hold you in my hands.

❀ Softly I bend my knees.

❀ I begin tilting my pelvis backwards and forwards, using the same movement as in the Cat sequence described in week 16. I arch my spine and open my chest (a) when I inhale and scoop my tailbone under, rounding my back, as I exhale (b).

❀ I practise this a few times.

❀ Then I begin to gently sway my hips from side to side. Keeping my spine straight, I take both my hips over to the right and then over to the left, repeating this several times on each side.

❀ Combining all four movements, I move like a belly dancer, circulating my hips and rotating my pelvis in a clockwise direction.

❀ I then repeat it all in an anticlockwise direction.

❀ I play some music and together we dance.

❀ I call it my birthing dance.

❀ Mindfully I repeat this week's affirmation:

My pelvis is designed to fit the shape of my baby's head.

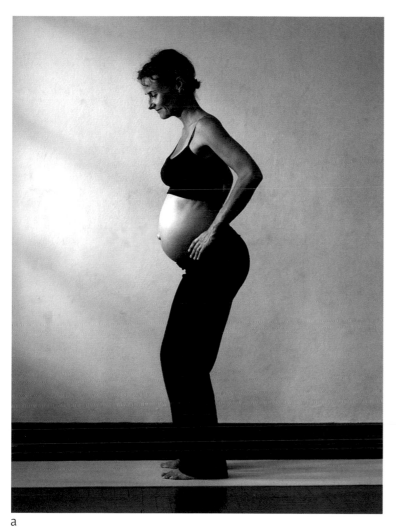

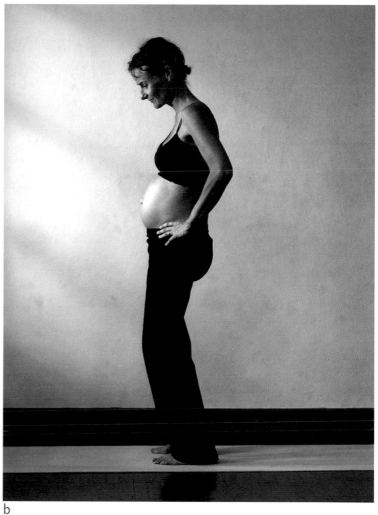

a

b

Reflection

Creating my own birthing dance,
I intuitively moved my body,
exercising and connecting with the most influential structure
of my body, specifically designed for childbirth,
the pelvis.

NAMASTÉ

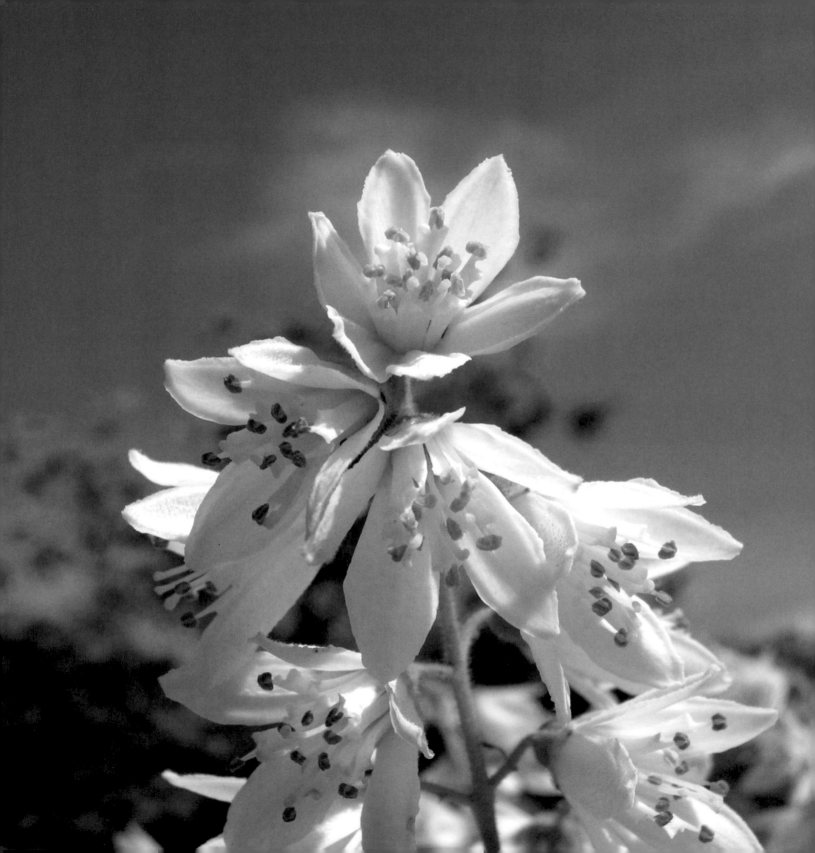

Our Eyes

*My baby's eyes are open
ready to receive the wonders of the world.*

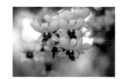

With a soft gaze I will look up, down, left and right, finding a focus to steady myself in a practice that honors one of the most delicate yet complex structures of the body: our eyes.

We are now in the final weeks of the second trimester.

While you put on weight, so do I. This reassures me that you are growing bigger and stronger.

Since you are increasingly sensitive to taste, you'll be pleased to hear that any cravings I had for strange concoctions in the early stages of pregnancy have finally left me and I find myself naturally avoiding very bitter, spicy or strong-tasting food.

Resisting the temptation of eating for two, I remind myself that what is healthy for me is healthy for you. Sharing with you all the goodness from my diet ensures that your placenta remains rich in nutrients and minerals to support you through these final stages of your development.

This week is dedicated to your eyes; the most complex and powerful sense. Up until now they have been carefully crafted under closed eyelids, but as your sensory development nears its completion the muscles of your eyes begin to blink and flicker awake and your eyes unveil themselves.

Although there isn't much for you to see in your uterine world, you become more sensitive to light and dark, night and day.

You will be born with blue eyes, until your irises define their final colour several months after your birth-day; I wonder what colour eyes you will inherit.

BENEFITS: *Anjaneyasana stretches the hips and upper thighs; strengthens the lower back and pelvic muscles; opens the chest; improves circulation and respiration.*

CAUTIONS: *I will avoid this pose if I have pelvic girdle discomfort.*

MODIFICATIONS: *If I have sensitive knees I will place a cushion under my back knee. To help steady myself or if I have high blood pressure I will practise the pose with my hands on my knees and look forward (b).*

Intention

I close my eyes.
Slowly blinking them open I look around
and imagine that I am seeing the world for the very first time.
With an 'I spy with my little eye',
I see endless, myriad images;
sizes, shapes and rainbow colours,
playing like a beautiful seamless movie before me.

Asana for the Week

Anjaneyasana – Crescent Moon

For this pose I will need a yoga mat and a small cushion.
   This pose is suitable for all stages of my pregnancy.

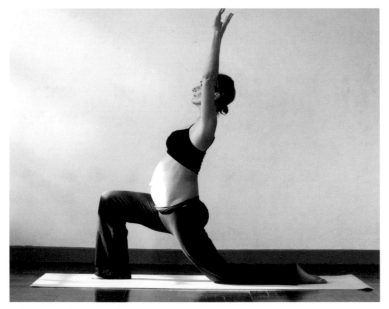

a Gaze at the thumbs

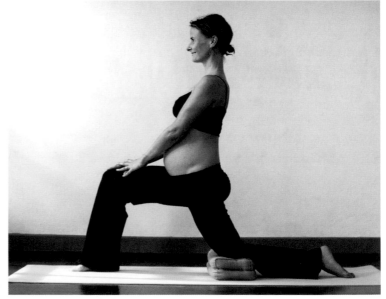

b Gaze straight ahead

❀ I come into a tabletop position and step my right foot in between my hands. I make room for you by shuffling my right foot over to the right. I look down to check my right knee is stacked directly over my right ankle and aligned with my second and third toes.

❀ I extend back and out through my left leg.

❀ I bring my torso upright so it stacks over my pelvis and glance at my hips to ensure that they are facing forward.

❀ I look down towards my belly and see it rising and falling with my breath.

❀ On an inhalation I reach my arms up over my head, and exhaling I soften my shoulders away from my ears.

❀ I softly gaze towards my hands (a).

❀ Staying for five breaths, I mindfully repeat this week's affirmation:

My baby's eyes are open,
ready to receive the wonders of the world.

❀ I repeat the pose to my other side.

Reflection

This week I used different foci in my practice
to help concentrate my mind, pause my thoughts,
and align my body as we gently exercised
our eyes.

NAMASTÉ

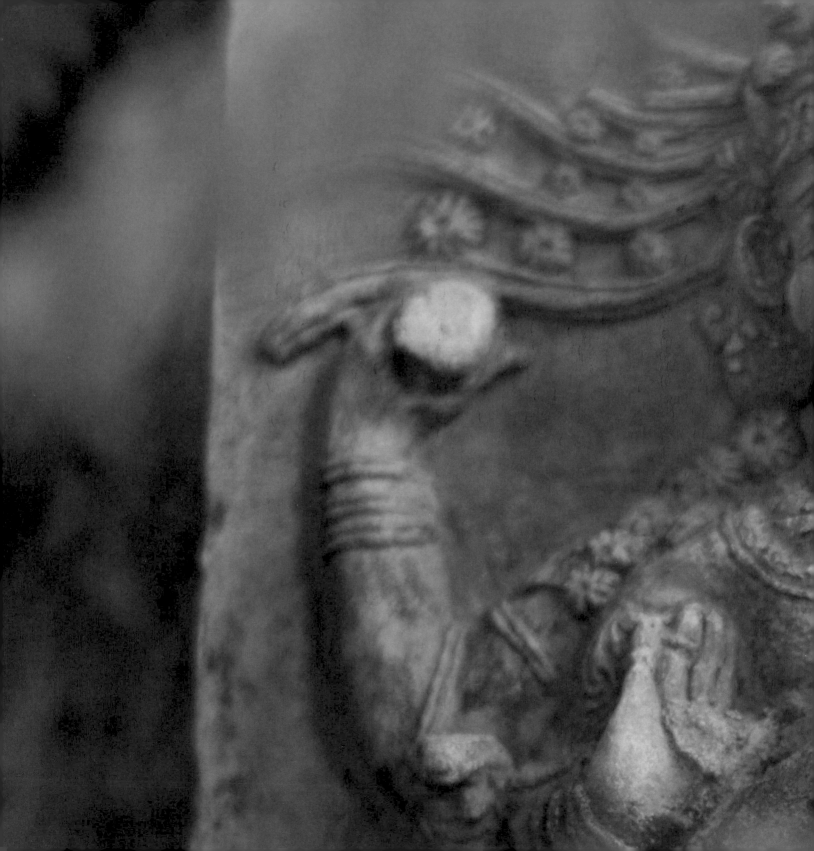

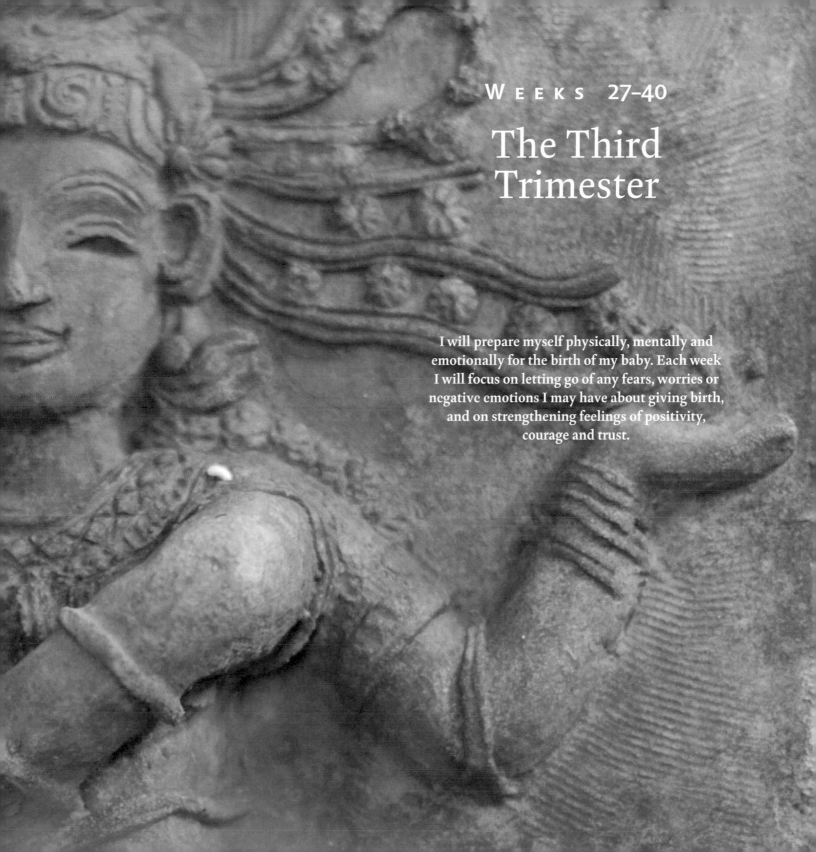

The Third Trimester

I will prepare myself physically, mentally and emotionally for the birth of my baby. Each week I will focus on letting go of any fears, worries or negative emotions I may have about giving birth, and on strengthening feelings of positivity, courage and trust.

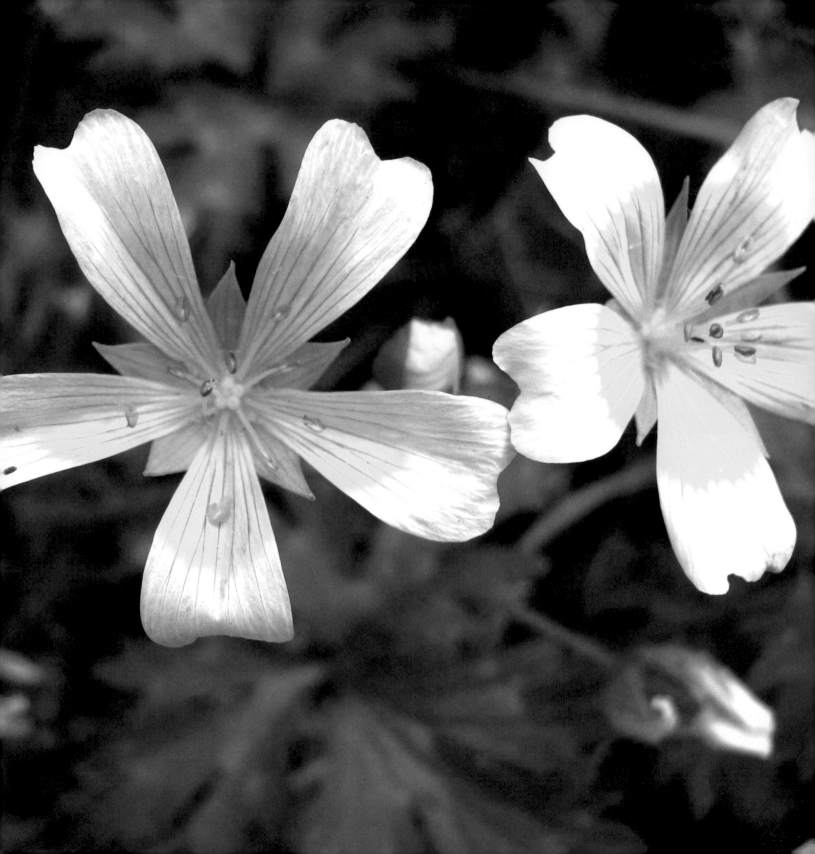

Stillness

I will be totally relaxed and at ease when I give birth to my baby.

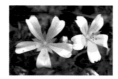

In full appreciation of all the changes taking place inside my body, I will take time this week to be with you in stillness.

You are now opening and closing your eyes, finding a rhythm to your sleeping patterns. They don't always coincide with mine; often it is when I am still that I notice that you are most active. Lying awake, sensitive to your wriggles, I imagine you trying to find a comfortable position to rest in, and attempting to suck your thumb. As well as being comforting, this is the perfect way to help strengthen your jaw and cheek muscles in preparation for you suckling later on.

Your lungs are developing steadily. Mine, however, become a little more squashed as my body makes room for you to grow. I am noticing how easily I become breathless now when doing everyday activities.

Regular gentle exercise is supporting my body and spirit though, and helps to keep my circulatory system fit and healthy.

As we enter the third trimester I find myself thinking more about your birth-day.

I am considering all the various options available to me: home birth, natural birth, the local hospital.

I want your birth-day to be a beautiful occasion for us both.

BENEFITS: *Supported Upavista Konasana stretches the inner thighs, hips and groin; relaxes the pelvic-floor muscles; lengthens the spine and releases tension in the lower back.*
It also helps to alleviate pelvic girdle discomfort symptoms.

Intention

Pressing the pause button in my daily life,
I will rest my body and mind.
I will invite silence between my words,
space between my thoughts
and stillness between my actions.

Asana for the Week

Supported Upavista Konasana

Supported Wide-Legged Forward Fold

For this pose I will need a yoga mat and several small cushions.
This pose is suitable for all stages of my pregnancy.

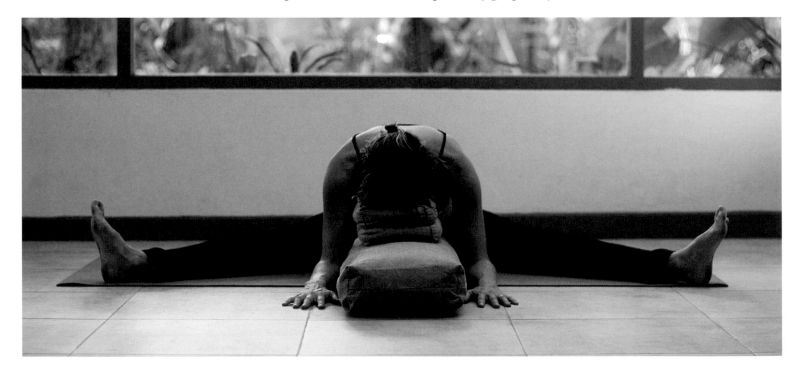

✿ I sit on my yoga mat with my legs gently stretched out to the sides. I stack some cushions and place them in between my legs. Tilting from my pelvis, I softly fold forward and rest my head on the cushions. My hands rest gently on the floor at either side. I invite stillness into my body and mind, simply enjoying being here with you.

✿ I bring my attention to my breath. I notice the natural pause at the end of my inhalation and at the end of my exhalation.

✿ I focus my mind on the pause at the end of my exhalations, allowing myself to drop into this stillness. I feel its depth and expanse as I immerse myself more fully, more completely into this pause.

✿ Staying here for up to ten minutes, I mindfully repeat this week's affirmation:

I will be totally relaxed and at ease when I give birth to my baby.

CAUTIONS: *If I have pelvic girdle discomfort I will bring my legs closer together, so they are only as wide as my outer hips.*

MODIFICATIONS: *If I experience discomfort in the backs of my knees I will bring my legs towards each other until the discomfort diminishes, and place a folded blanket under my knees.*
To allow more room for you, as my pregnancy progresses I can use a bed or the seat of a chair to rest my head on.

Reflection

In my practice I found peace in my body and mind,
uniting with you in
stillness.

NAMASTÉ

WEEK 28

Mindfulness

*The sensory and neurological pathways are communicating with each other,
preparing my growing baby to become a conscious being of the world.*

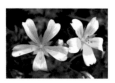

I will become a witness to my thoughts and simply allow them to pass by in the presence of mindfulness.

The architecture of your brain continues to develop, with new hills and valleys, grooves and ridges, its previous smooth appearance slowly disappearing.

The dynamics of your nervous system are rapidly becoming more refined, with the fatty protective layer of myelin continuing to cloak your billions of nerve fibers so they can send messages at a faster rate.

You are becoming more sensitive and responsive to light, touch, sound and taste; sometimes you signal your likes and dislikes of the food we share with a little somersault or hiccup.

Each day I try to spend special time reading, singing or talking to you.

Consciously sending you positive thoughts and messages of affirmations to reassure you that all is well as I start to make plans and prepare for your birth-day.

Although my belly is expanding with your weight gain, your home is becoming a little cramped and there is less room for you to move around.

Your once gentle flutterings are turning into more assertive kicks; sometimes they even take my breath away and I have to stop what I'm doing.

I wish I felt as agile and energetic as you!

Intention

This week I will enrich my diet with a variety of brain-food ingredients. I will fuel our nervous systems and strengthen our brain cells with fresh fruit, leafy green vegetables and food rich in essential fatty acids, which support our memory and keep our minds fit and healthy.

Asana for the Week

Baddha Konasana – Bound Angle Pose

For this pose I will need a yoga mat and several small cushions.
   This pose is suitable for all stages of my pregnancy.

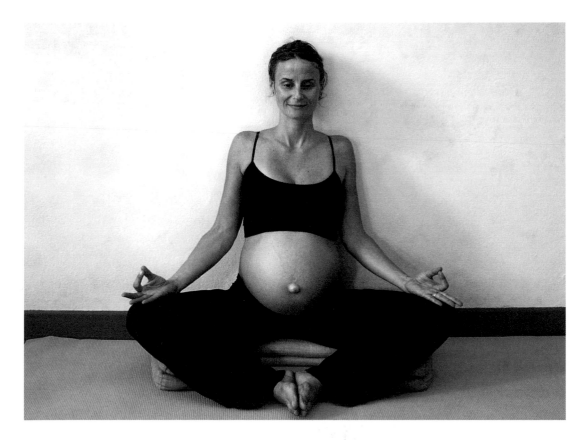

BENEFITS: *Baddha Konasana stretches the inner thighs, hips and groin; relaxes the pelvic-floor muscles; lengthens the spine and releases tension in the lower back.*

CAUTIONS: *If I have pelvic girdle discomfort I will practise the Birthing Breath sitting on my heels with my knees together, and place a cushion(s) between my sitting bones and my heels to bridge any gaps.*

MODIFICATIONS: *If my knees are higher than my hips as I sit in this pose, I will place a cushion(s) under my sitting bones to create a downward slope in my thighs. I will also slide my heels further away from my perineum to create a larger diamond shape. If needed, I will place a cushion(s) under my thighs to fully support me in the pose.*

❀ I sit on several cushions with my back against the wall. I bring the soles of my feet together to create a diamond shape between my perineum and my heels. I place a cushion under each knee to help my legs relax into this shape.

❀ I rest the backs of my hands on my thighs, bringing the tip of each thumb to the tip of the index finger while extending my other three fingers. This hand gesture is Jnana mudra, which symbolizes the uniting of our unconscious with our conscious energy.

❀ I think of you growing into a new conscious being, becoming sensitive and expressive within your world.

❀ I become mindful of my breath pattern and begin to practice the Birthing Breath as described in week 18 (see pages 63/64).

❀ Mindfully I repeat this week's affirmation:

> *The sensory and neurological pathways are communicating with each other,*
> *preparing my growing baby to become a conscious being of the world.*

❀ Gradually my breath settles back into its natural rhythm.

Reflection

This week I connected with my breath to help relax my mind,
pause my thoughts, and gently ease my body into a practice of
mindfulness.

NAMASTÉ

WEEK 29

Courage

Each powerful surge is my body's way of bringing my baby closer to me.

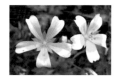

I will seek the qualities of a warrior in this practice; perseverance, endurance, confidence and courage.

This final chapter of my pregnancy is one of rapid growth for you and I find comfort in seeing my belly expand, knowing that you are putting on weight and getting stronger in preparation for your life outside my womb.

Your skeletal system continues to harden and lengthen. Your muscles are strengthening with your repetitive and dynamic movements and your head is growing in proportion to your maturing brain.

My belly is clearly rounded now, expanding from underneath my ribcage to my pubis. Some days I feel energetic like you, and other days I feel breathless and fatigued.

Sometimes my digestion feels a little sluggish and I get constipated. I remember the practice of Prasarita Padottanasana from the beginning of the second trimester, which can help to get things moving again (see page 46).

Sporadically I experience feelings of tightening or squeezing across my abdomen. These are known as Braxton Hicks contractions. This is my uterus contracting, rehearsing for our big day.

When I feel one of these early contractions, I imagine giving you a gentle hug from the inside. I wonder if you feel it too as you now are more sensitive to everything happening around you.

BENEFITS: *Virabhadrasana II stretches the hamstrings, hips and calves; strengthens the thighs and lengthens the spine.*

CAUTIONS: *It is advised that I do not practise deep or unsupported squats after week 34 of my pregnancy or once my baby is engaged.*
I can continue to practise this pose by straddling a chair with my right sitting bone and the top of my right thigh resting on the seat of the chair, then repeating the pose to my other side.
I will avoid this pose if I have pelvic girdle discomfort.

MODIFICATIONS: *If I have high blood pressure it is advised that I practise this pose with my hands on my hips.*

Intention

This week, I will use my breath as an instrumental key.
On an inhalation I will invite myself to step inside
and open the doors to faith, patience, endurance and courage.
On an exhalation I will unlock any tension, worries or fears I may be holding onto.
Using my breath I will soften, relax and surrender,
and visualize the birth-day I desire.

Asana for the Week

Virabhadrasana II – Warrior 2

For this pose I will need a yoga mat and a wall or a chair.

❀ Placing my yoga mat against a wall, I take a wide stance with my feet facing forward and parallel to each other. I feel the support of the wall behind me.

❀ I turn my right foot out, aligning my right heel with the middle of the arch of my left foot.

❀ I wrap my arms around you and check that both of my hips are facing into the center of the room.

❀ Feeling my expanding belly I instinctively look down at you and smile.

❀ I take a breath.

❀ Inhaling, I raise my arms up and out to the side so they are in line with my shoulders. I look out towards my right fingers.

❀ Exhaling, I bend my right knee, stacking it directly above my ankles, and aligning it with my second and third toes.

❀ While in this pose I think of the structure of my body and the strength of my muscles holding me here and I think of you.

❀ I feel bold, strong and courageous like a warrior, as I begin to prepare myself mentally for your birth.

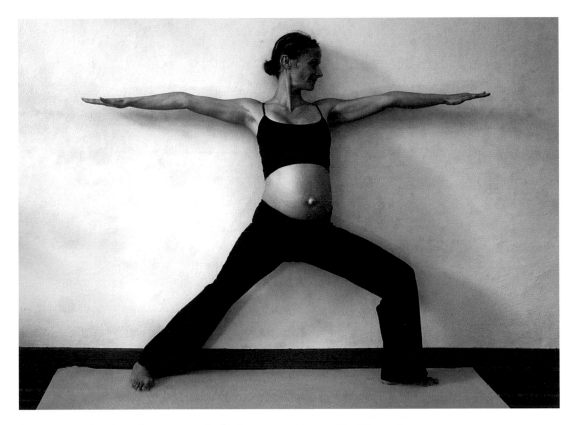

❀ Staying for three breaths, I mindfully repeat this week's affirmation:

Each powerful surge is my body's way of bringing my baby closer to me.

❀ I repeat the pose to my other side.

Reflection

*Committed to a fearless and positive attitude
towards the birth of my baby, this week's practice was an expression of our
resounding strength, determination and courage.*

NAMASTÉ

WEEK 30

Empowerment

I am in control of making the right decisions to have the right birth for me and my baby.

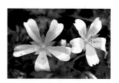

I visualize the birth I desire and nurture the power from within to create a spirit of empowerment.

As I begin to plan and get ready for your arrival, you too are busy, making your own preparations to help equip yourself for the outside world.

Your digestive, circulatory and respiratory systems are now fully functioning and you are starting to regulate your own body temperature, thanks to all the fatty layers you have been developing underneath your skin to protect and keep you warm.

As you are steadily putting on fat, there is less room for you to stretch out and somersault and I notice that your movements are a little more forceful. At times I find myself watching my skin undulate, feeling the presence of you writhing around.

I enjoy having fun trying to guess which part of your body is reaching out; a smooth rump I guess to be your back or bottom, and a pointed protrusion perhaps your elbow or knee. I design a map in my mind of where you lie in my belly.

You are my little yogini.

Intention

*I become empowered with positive thoughts,
reminding myself that I am a strong, capable woman
who has the strength, resilience and knowledge
to give birth to my baby with ease and grace.*

Asana for the Week

Parsvakonasana – Standing Side Angle Stretch

For this pose I will need a yoga mat, a wall or a chair.

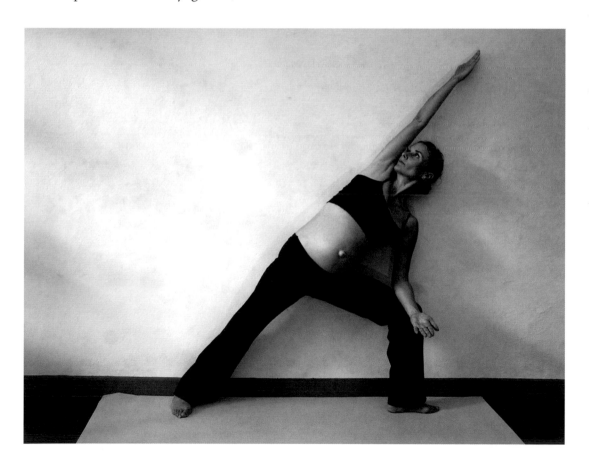

BENEFITS: *Parsvakonasana
stretches the shoulders, chest,
hamstrings, hips and calves;
strengthens the thighs and
improves stamina.*

CAUTIONS: *It is advised that I do
not practise deep or unsupported
squats after week 34 of my
pregnancy or once my baby is
engaged.
I can continue to practise this
pose by straddling a chair with my
right sitting bone and the top of
my right thigh resting on the seat
of the chair, then repeating the
pose on my other side.
I will avoid this pose if I have
pelvic girdle discomfort.*

MODIFICATIONS: *If I have high
blood pressure it is advised that I
practise this pose with my raised
arm on my hip instead.*

❀ Placing my yoga mat against a wall, I take the shape of Virabhadrasana II from last week's practice (see page 103).

❀ Softening down through my right thigh, I extend my upper body over to the right. I bend my right elbow and rest it on my right thigh with my palm facing up. I bring my left hand to rest on you.

❀ I wonder if I will feel you move as you make shapes with your body too.

❀ When I feel ready I raise my left arm up and over to rest next to my left ear.

❀ I can choose between looking forward or turning my gaze up towards my left hand.

❀ Staying for three breaths, I mindfully repeat this week's affirmation:

*I am in control of making the right decisions to
have the right birth for me and my baby.*

❀ I repeat the pose to my other side.

Reflection

*To help me prepare for labor
I have learnt to move my body safely and intuitively,
affirm positive thoughts, use my voice constructively,
focus on my breath and cultivate feelings of
empowerment.*

NAMASTÉ

Rest and Revive

It is important that I rest whenever I can during these final weeks of pregnancy, to help me prepare my mind, body and soul to give birth to my baby.

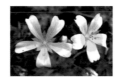

To help prepare myself for your birth-day, it is important that I listen to my body's needs, conserve my energy and gather my strength, taking any opportunity I can to rest and revive.

You are maturing and growing at an astonishing rate now, adding weight daily.

Your respiratory system continues to develop. While your chest wall and diaphragm refine their structures ready to help support the mechanics of your breathing, your lungs have still to reach full maturity.

The alveoli in your lungs continue to unfold and branch out and a greasy substance, called surfactant, masks the interior of your lungs to protect them and help you breathe with ease once you are born.

Steadily your immune system gains strength, strength that I hope to complement with breast-feeding you once you are born. My breasts are becoming noticeably fuller and sometimes leak colostrum, a sign that my body is preparing for your arrival. This first milk, sometimes referred to as 'Liquid Gold', is what I will feed you when you are first born; it contains a yummy collection of natural antibiotics, probiotics and stem cells to quench your thirsty appetite and support your immune system.

While my body prepares itself for your birth-day, I should take rest during the day whenever I can; the physical demands that giving birth will place on my body can be compared to running a marathon!

BENEFITS: *Supported Reclining Twist with a bolster improves breathing and circulation; relieves tension in the shoulders and back muscles and calms the mind.*

CAUTIONS: *I will discontinue practising this pose if it becomes uncomfortable for me. I will let my body be my guide.*

MODIFICATIONS: *As my pregnancy progresses I will use additional cushions, placing one between my thighs and one under my belly to make the pose more comfortable for me and to provide extra support for my growing baby.*

Intention

As I lie on my left side and relax,
I will meditate upon the rhythm of my breath.
I will remind myself that for the next few minutes
there is nothing to do, nowhere to go.
I will simply allow myself to be;
Not doing or thinking,
just being ... with you.

Asana for the Week

Supported Reclining Twist

For this pose I will need a yoga mat, a bolster or long pillow and a folded blanket. This pose is suitable for all stages of my pregnancy.

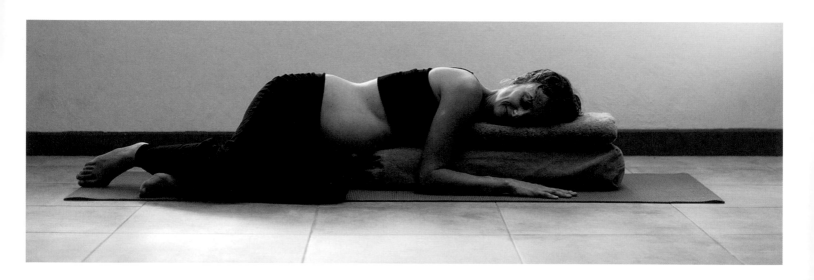

❀ Sitting on my yoga mat, I place the short end of my long cushion or bolster against my right hip, placing a folded blanket at the other end.

❀ Bending my knees, I slide my legs over to the left, then rest my hands on the floor either side of my bolster and turn my upper chest to the right. I walk my hands forward, extending and resting my torso over the bolster. I relax the right side of my head on the blanket. My arms rest softly on the floor beside me.

❀ I welcome my breath, surrendering deeper into the pose with each breath. Letting go of my thoughts, I enjoy some quiet moments of not doing, simply being here with you and taking time to restore my energy.

❀ Staying here for three to five minutes, I mindfully repeat this week's affirmation:

> *It is important that I rest whenever I can during these final weeks of pregnancy,*
> *to help me prepare my mind, body and soul to give birth to my baby.*

❀ I repeat the pose to my other side.

❀ To come out of the pose I remove the bolster, bend my knees and rest on my left side. I stay here for a few minutes before using my hands to gently assist me up into a sitting position.

Reflection

To help prepare myself for the birth of my baby,
I relaxed and restored my mind, body and soul
in a peaceful practice that encouraged me to
rest and revive.

NAMASTÉ

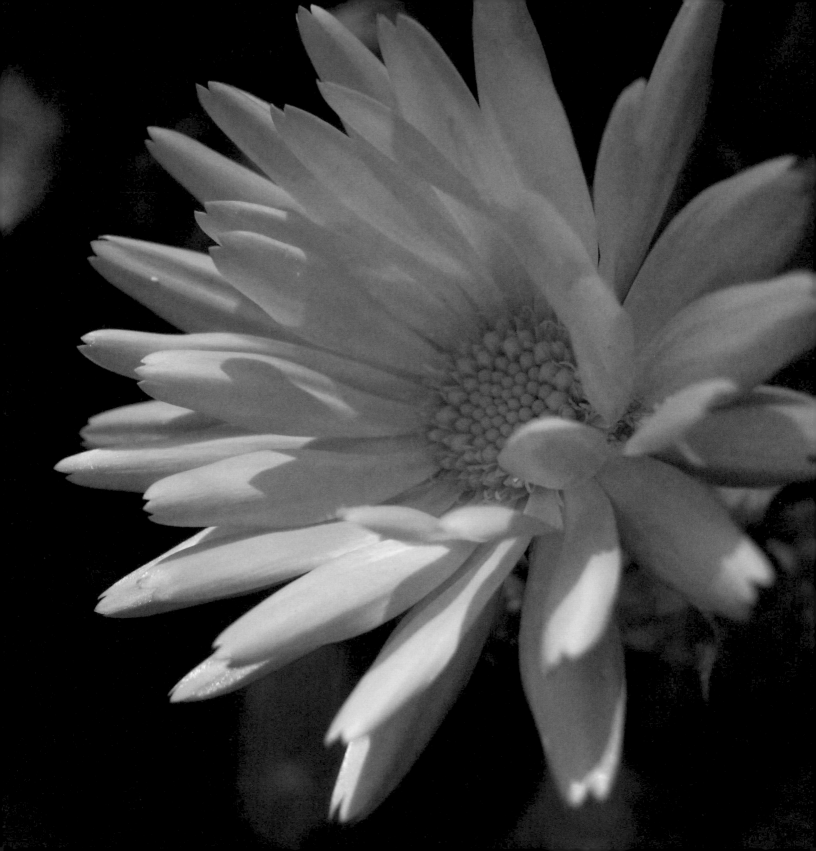

WEEK 32

Flexibility

This labor is my labor and the right one for me and my baby.

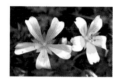

I will learn to accept, respond and adapt to new and challenging situations by practising flexibility.

You now resemble a newborn. You have the body of a perfectly formed little person and your skin is changing from translucent to a warm shade of pink.

The downy fine hair, lanugo, that lightly decorates your skin is beginning to moult; however, you still remain cloaked in the waxy substance vernix caseosa, which protects your skin and insulates you to keep you warm as you lie bathed in my amniotic fluid.

This protective coat will also help you to slide with relative ease along the birth canal on your birth-day.

Your head may now be starting to try to nestle, like a perfectly fitting puzzle, into my pelvis.

If you're not there yet, no need to worry; there is still plenty of time to twist and turn to find that comfortable place to rest in readiness for your delivery into my world.

Stay inside your cozy uterine home just a little longer; you are safe there and I am reassured by your constant movements that all is well – sometimes I find myself counting them and there can be as many as ten per hour!

BENEFITS: *Marichyasana III Twist Variation improves digestion and elimination; strengthens and lengthens the spine, helps relieve back tension; stretches the shoulders and chest; calms the mind and helps balance emotions.*

MODIFICATIONS: *To help maintain length in my spine and prevent rounding in my lower back I will use the support of a cushion under my sitting bones and I will use a block to rest my back hand on (b).*

Intention

*Finalizing your birth-day arrangements this week,
I will note down all my birth plan wishes.
I will practise flexibility of the mind;
to be adaptable and open to change.
Accepting any differences with grace and dignity,
I will respond in a loving, intelligent
and soulful way.*

Asana for the Week

Marichyasana III – Twist Variation: Sage Open Twist

For this pose I will need a yoga mat, a small cushion and a block. This pose is suitable for all stages of my pregnancy.

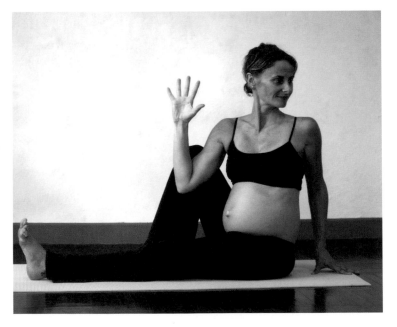
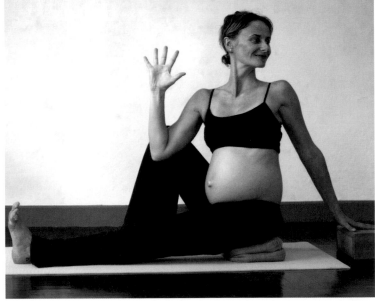

❀ I sit on my yoga mat with my legs straight out in front of me, making sure you have space I separate my legs so they are slightly wider than my hips. I bend my right knee and place my right foot in line with my left knee.

❀ I shuffle my right foot over to the right edge of my mat to make room for you and ensure we are both comfortable.

❀ I sit up tall, lengthening my spine.

❀ Bending my right elbow, I rest it against the inside of my right knee.

❀ My left hand rests on the floor behind me in line with my left sitting bone (a).

❀ I turn my heart center to the left. I remind myself that when situations arise that feel twisted, distorted or out of sorts I need to come back into my center and take a look from a different angle in order to see things with a clearer perception.

❀ Staying for three breaths, I mindfully repeat this week's affirmation:

This labor is my labor and the right one for me and my baby.

❀ I repeat the pose to my other side.

Reflection

By accepting the physical and emotional changes in pregnancy, I have learnt to open my body and mind in different ways to find flexibility.

NAMASTÉ

Positivity

Each powerful sensation in labor is nature's way of bringing my baby to me.

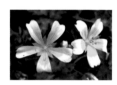

I will visualize the birth I desire, replace negative thoughts with affirmations and use my practice to express feelings of positivity.

Squashed together, my organs rearrange themselves to make room for you in my growing uterus, which has now inflated to several times its normal size. Providing you with the perfect home, my body continues to supply you with all the ongoing nourishment and protection you need to complete your journey of creation.

You have now filled out and have adorable chubby little arms and legs.

I, on the other hand, feel cumbersome and large; I am still getting used to my changing shape and new body image.

Waddling around, I notice that I can no longer squeeze behind counters or slide in between people – I need more room for the two of us.

Looking down, though, I can still see my toes to check for any signs of swelling, and as my centre of gravity perpetually changes, regular exercise and yoga is helping me to maintain a good posture and fend off any lower-back discomfort.

For the past seven months we have shared so many intimate moments, and I am overwhelmed by this enduring, deep love I feel for you.

Intention

Idly I daydream and paint a picture of your birth-day.
I see myself using my breath to remain calm and composed with each surge,
and instinctively moving to the inner callings from my body.
Casting my thoughts to you I see you in my mind's eye,
entering the world with ease.
I hold on to this image, affirming it with positive thoughts,
to help prepare my mind, body and soul
for your birth-day.

Asana for the Week

Thai Goddess Pose

For this pose I will need a yoga mat and a small cushion(s).
   This pose is suitable for all stages of my pregnancy.

❁ I place my yoga mat against a wall and move into a tabletop position with my heels resting up against the wall. I curl my toes under and sit back on my heels, using a cushion(s) to bridge any gaps between my sitting bones and heels. I rest my upper back against the wall and bring my hands together in front of my heart center in the gesture of a loving touch, Anjali mudra.

❁ I am aware of discomfort in my toes while I am in the Thai Goddess Pose, but I practise replacing any negative feelings I have with positive ones, focusing on my breath and using sound to help calm my mind.

❁ I practise the Birthing Breath, for five breaths (see pages 63–6).

❁ As I feel the discomfort of the pose intensifying I imagine it to be a surge reaching its peak. I inhale through my nose and exhale through my mouth, directing my out-breath down to you and my pelvic floor. I remember to smile.

❁ Returning to tabletop position, I uncurl my toes and take ten natural breaths.

BENEFITS: Thai Goddess Pose gives a strong stretch to the soles of the feet; this is the intention, however, use it as an opportunity to practise the Birthing Breath and make deep vowel sounds to surrender into the stretch and help ease the discomfort.
The Birthing Breath and deep vowel sounds can be valuable tools in labor to help direct the energy down to the base of the body and help to relax the pelvic-floor muscles to ease delivery.

CAUTIONS: I will avoid this pose if I have knee injuries; however I will still continue to practise the Birthing Breath.

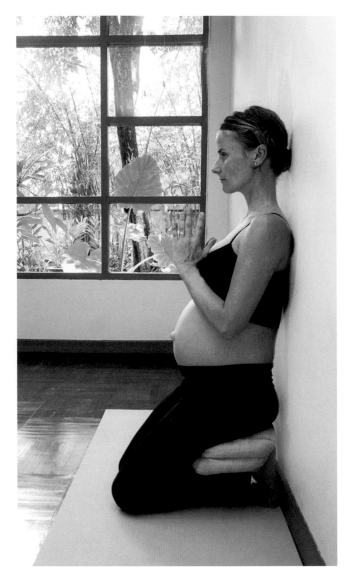

❀ Mindfully I repeat this week's affirmation:

Each powerful sensation in labor is nature's way of bringing my baby to me.

❀ Returning to the Thai Goddess Pose I sound the vowel "ooo" along with my exhalation. I practise this five times, then ease out of the pose, take ten natural breaths.

❀ I repeat the pose and sound the vowel "aaahhh" five times.

❀ I concentrate on replacing any negative feelings I have with positive ones, focusing on my breath and using sound to help calm my mind. I come out of the pose and slowly allow my breath to return to its natural rhythm.

Reflection

This week I was encouraged to erase any negative thoughts or emotions I may have surrounding the birth of my baby and instead nurture feelings of inner peace, strength and positivity.

NAMASTÉ

WEEK 34

Gratitude

Thank you for being my baby.

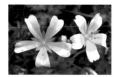

Cultivating feelings of thankfulness, I will bow to my heart and find ways to express my feelings of gratitude.

You are now almost like a newborn baby.

Your internal system is almost fully functioning, just awaiting the finishing touches to your liver, kidneys and lungs.

The millions of connections within your nervous system are communicating, responding and interacting with your mind and body.

You have established a rhythm to your sleeping patterns and you respond to touch, taste, sound and light.

The hair on your head is growing and the wrinkles on your skin smoothing themselves out, effortlessly disappearing as you fill out.

I hope they weren't worry lines – there is no need to worry, my little one, we are almost there!

Your skin acts like a quilt, keeping you warm and safe, and your complexion becomes a shade of rosy pink.

Each day you are becoming more beautiful as you get ready for your birth-day.

BENEFITS: *Ardha Parsvottanasana stretches the hamstrings, hips and calves; strengthens the thighs and lengthens the spine.*

MODIFICATIONS: *To help steady myself I will position a chair in front of me to hold on to (b) or I will practise the pose facing a wall, keeping my spine and arms straight and resting my palms against the wall.*

Intention

I will look inside my heart and silently recite an invocation of gratitude.
I will thank my body for providing a safe haven for you to grow.
I will give thanks to the miracle of life,
and to all the great gifts it has given me.
I will give thanks to all the people who share their love,
guidance and support with our journey,
and I thank you for choosing me to be your mother.

Asana for the Week

Ardha Parsvottanasana – Half Intense Side Stretch Pose

For this pose I will need a yoga mat and a chair or a wall to help steady myself. This pose is suitable for all stages of my pregnancy.

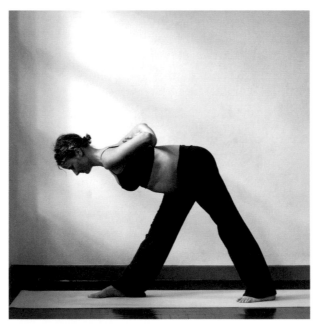

a

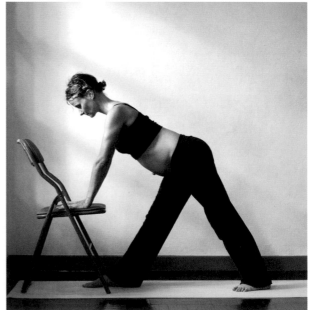

b

❀ Standing at the top of my yoga mat, I step my left foot back and turn it out at a slight angle. I align my hips and chest to face forward.

❀ Grounding down through my left heel, I inhale and lengthen my spine. As I exhale I tilt from my hips and extend my torso forward. I bring my arms behind my back and hold on to each forearm with the opposite hand (a).

❀ As I bow into this pose, serenity fills my soul. I feel at peace with my world. Looking down at my front foot, I glance towards you and see my beautiful belly.

❀ Staying for three breaths, I mindfully repeat this week's affirmation:

Thank you for being my baby.

❀ I repeat the pose to my other side.

Reflection

This week I simply said thank you in a practice that was filled with appreciation and overflowing with sentiments of gratitude.

NAMASTÉ

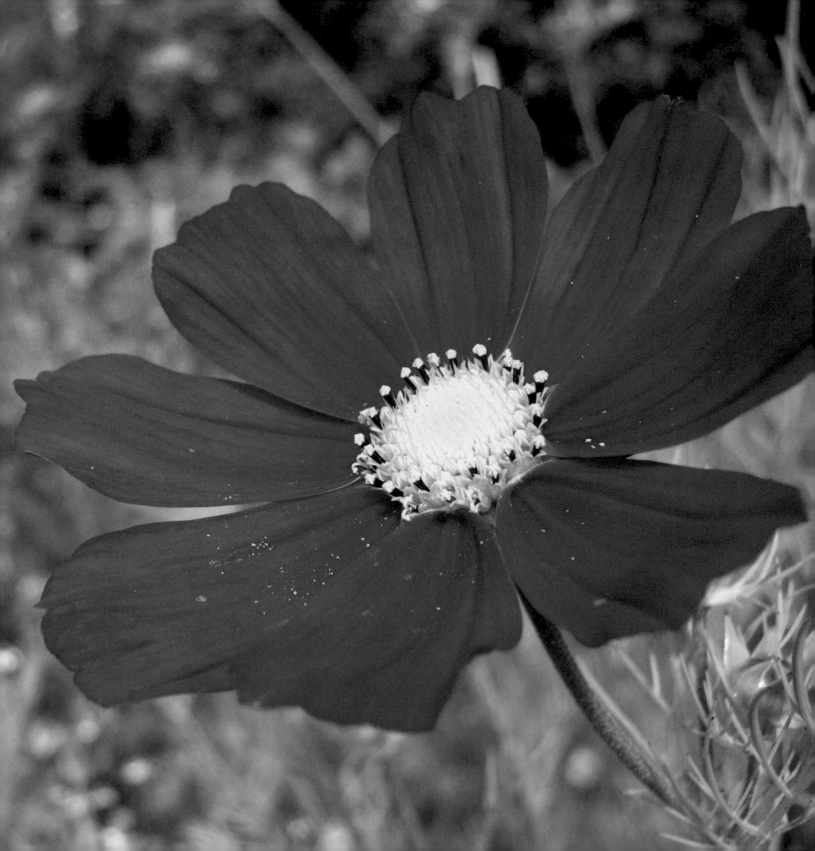

WEEK 35

Patience

When my baby is ready they will have their birth-day.

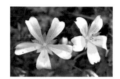

As I expectantly prepare for the arrival of my new baby, it is important that I rest, conserve my energy and remind myself of the virtue of having patience.

As your birth-day comes closer, we are both preparing for your arrival in our own special ways.

While I prepare my home for you, making sure you will have a comfortable place to rest, feed and play, you are busy priming yourself for a safe passage into this world.

Your waxy coat, the vernix caseosa, is thickening to give your skin a slippery film and although your bones have hardened, the ones inside your skull remain soft and pliable to help you ease your way down the birth canal into my world.

This week your liver and kidneys finalize their development and their roles in elimination.

Waste products are now being stored in your intestine; meconium, a green sticky tar-like substance, will be your first bowel movements when you are born.

As this final period is one of rapid growth for you, I am ensuring that my diet contains plenty of nutrients to give us both strength for your birth-day.

When I can, I like to snuggle up with you and dream of our beautiful love affair. Holding you in my arms I rock you to sleep with the sweet lullaby of my heartbeat.

BENEFITS: *Supta Baddha Konasana stretches the inner thighs, hips and groin; relaxes the pelvic-floor muscles; opens the upper chest; improves breathing; lengthens the spine and releases tension in the lower back.*

CAUTIONS: *If I have pelvic girdle discomfort I will practise the Supported Reclining Pose as described on pages 29/30. I will discontinue practising this pose if it becomes uncomfortable for me. I will let my body be my guide.*

Intention

*This week I will put aside my to-do list
and enjoy some precious moments being with you.
Counting down the days until your birth-day,
I will practise being patient.*

Asana for the Week

Supta Baddha Konasana – Reclined Bound Angle Pose

For this pose I will need a yoga mat, a bolster or long pillow, a folded blanket, several small cushions to support my back, legs and arms, and an eye pillow.

    This pose is suitable for all stages of my pregnancy.

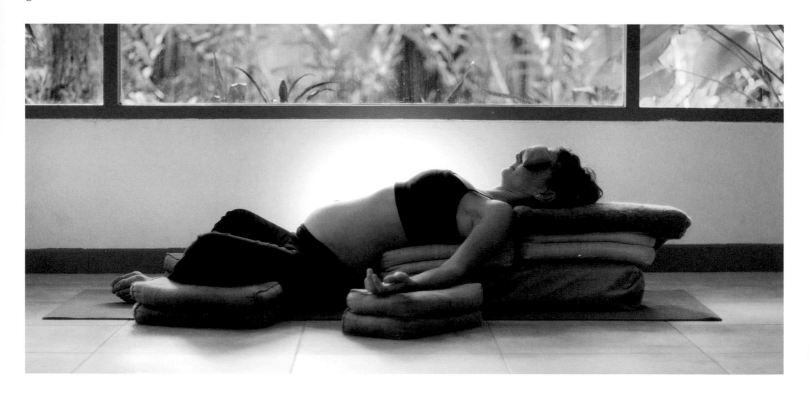

✳ I sit on my yoga mat surrounded by cushions. I place the short end of a bolster or long pillow behind me, snug to my lower back. I stack some cushions on top to create a semi-reclined 'chaise longue' shape for me to rest over.

✳ I place a folded blanket at the other end of my bolster, on which I will rest my head.

✳ Bringing the soles of my feet together, I form the shape of Baddha Konasana (see pages 99/100) and rest some cushions underneath my knees so my legs can relax and hips and groin open.

✳ I recline back over the bolster and cushions, and rest my head on the folded blanket.

✳ I ensure that my back is comfortable, making any adjustments I need to, finding the optimum position to rest in.

✳ I place an eye pillow over my eyes and let my arms rest on cushions at the sides of my body.

✳ I merge into the rhythm of my breath.

✳ By relinquishing any temptations to think or do, I learn to surrender, listen and focus on being present with you, which requires my patience.

✳ Staying here for up to ten minutes, I mindfully repeat this week's affirmation:

When my baby is ready they will have their birth-day.

✳ Afterwards I remove my eye pillow, bend my knees and roll over to my left side. I stay here for a few minutes before using my hands to gently assist me up into a sitting position.

Reflection

This week I took time to rest,
conserved my energy and surrendered into a practice of patience.

NAMASTÉ

WEEK 36

Intuition

I trust my body and my baby to know exactly what to do.

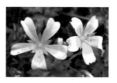

This week I will move my body instinctively to the natural rhythm of my breath and be guided by my own intuition.

After this week, you are classed as full-term.

All your organs, bones, muscles, tissues and senses are developed, your lungs requiring just a few more days to fully mature.

As you descend towards my pelvis, trying to find a comfy spot to settle and become fully engaged ready for your birth-day, I can sense a feeling of lightening. My stomach and lungs become less squashed and I find it more comfortable to eat and easier to breathe.

You do put a little added pressure on my bladder though, and visits to the bathroom are more frequent. Now I realize the importance of keeping up with my Kegel exercises!

While you happily continue to put on weight with untamed abandonment, my weight gain is steadying now.

Over the last nine months, both our bodies have undergone such phenomenal changes.

We are both now gorgeously round and beautiful, having blossomed into this final stage of pregnancy.

Intention

*During this pregnancy I have become increasingly
aware of my body and mindful of my baby's needs.
In labor I will take these gifts with me.
I will remain sensitive to each sensation,
follow my instincts, breathe
and listen to how my body and baby
wish for me to move.*

Asana for the Week

Seated Namasté Flow

For this pose I will need a yoga mat and a small cushion(s).
  This pose is suitable for all stages of my pregnancy.

❀ I find a comfortable cross-legged sitting position and bring my hands together in Anjali mudra in front of my heart. Bowing down towards my hands, I take a moment to set my intention for my practice (a).

❀ Mindfully I repeat this week's affirmation:

> *I trust my body and my baby to know exactly what to do.*

❀ Inhaling, I extend my arms out to the side (b), visualizing myself gathering up my innate wisdom and yours. I bring my hands to meet above my head and take my gaze towards my hands (c).

❀ Exhaling, I slowly bring my hands back in front of my heart. Following my hands with my gaze, I imagine this wisdom cascading into my soul and flowing down to you.

❀ I bow towards my hands, honoring this innate wisdom deep inside us (a).

❀ Mindfully I repeat this week's affirmation:

> *I trust my body and my baby to know exactly what to do.*

❀ I repeat this sequence five times, synchronizing the movements with my breath.

BENEFITS: *Seated Namasté Flow strengthens and stretches the shoulders; opens the chest; releases the hips; improves circulation and focuses and calms the mind.*

CAUTIONS: *If I have pelvic girdle discomfort I will do this practice sitting on my heels with my knees together. I will place a cushion(s) between my sitting bones and my heels to bridge any gaps.*

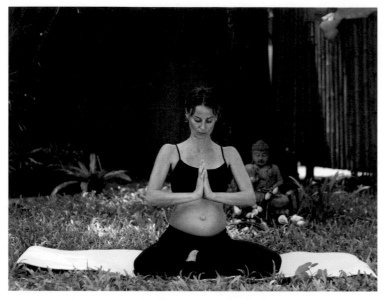

a

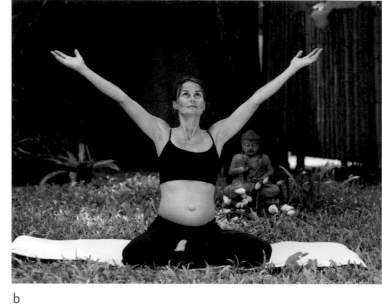

b

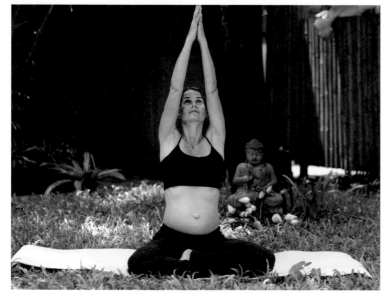

c

Reflection

By instinctively moving my body with the flow of my breath
I tuned in to my inner wisdom and listened to my intuition.

NAMASTÉ

WEEK 37

Contemplation

I deserve to have the birth of my dreams.

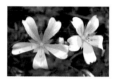

As I think about meeting you I will gather my pregnancy photographs, scans and memories of our journey together over the past nine months, taking time this week for some contemplation.

Congratulations, you are now reaching the end of your journey.

All your organs have now developed – this week marks the coming to maturity of your lungs.

Before long you will experience your first breath, taking in the air of the outside world and finding your own unique and natural rhythm.

For now, though, you continue to breathe with a special fluid made by your lungs and ingest the water of life, my amniotic fluid, practising your newly acquired skills of peeing, sleeping, breathing and feeding, and refine the skill of suckling by sucking your thumb.

Very soon you will learn to synchronize sucking and swallowing with breathing, a skill you will need once you begin to feed from me.

With your birth-day imminent, my body is getting ready for this special day. The mucus plug, which has acted like a protective seal to my cervix, might start to slowly come free in the form of a discharge, a signal that you may be on your way and that my cervix can get ready to dilate.

Take your time; it is safe for you to stay inside your uterine hideaway for another couple of weeks.

There is no rush.

BENEFITS: *Balasana stretches the inner thighs, hips and groin; relaxes the pelvic-floor muscles; lengthens the spine; releases tension in the lower back. Child's Pose can be a useful pose to rest in between surges during the early stages of labor, offering you respite and an opportunity to gather strength and resilience ready for the rising of the next surge.*

CAUTIONS: *If I have pelvic girdle discomfort or find this posture uncomfortable, I will come on to all fours into a tabletop position and use a birthing ball or the seat of a chair to rest my arms and head on.*

MODIFICATIONS: *If I experience discomfort in my knees I will place a cushion behind each knee.*

Intention

*This week I will recall our journey over the past nine months,
remembering this precious time we have spent together
living and breathing together,
entwined within each other's body.
I will keep each twist, turn, kick, hiccup
and Braxton Hicks squeeze etched on my memory,
 savoring all these wonderful sensations of carrying you inside me.*

Asana for the Week

Balasana – Child's Pose

For this pose I will need a yoga mat and several small cushions.
    This pose is suitable for all stages of my pregnancy.

❀   I come on to all fours into a tabletop position, taking my knees out wide to the sides and bringing my big toes to touch behind me. I sit back on my heels, using a cushion(s) to bridge any gaps between my sitting bones and heels.

❀   Tilting from my hips, I extend my torso and bow down. I walk my hands forward and rest my head on a cushion(s), making sure you have room to enjoy this pose too.

❀   Resting in Child's Pose, I will think about you, my child. I will reflect on our journey together so far and all that we have achieved. I will contemplate our lives ahead as mother and child.

❀   Staying for ten breaths, I mindfully repeat this week's affirmation:

I deserve to have the birth of my dreams.

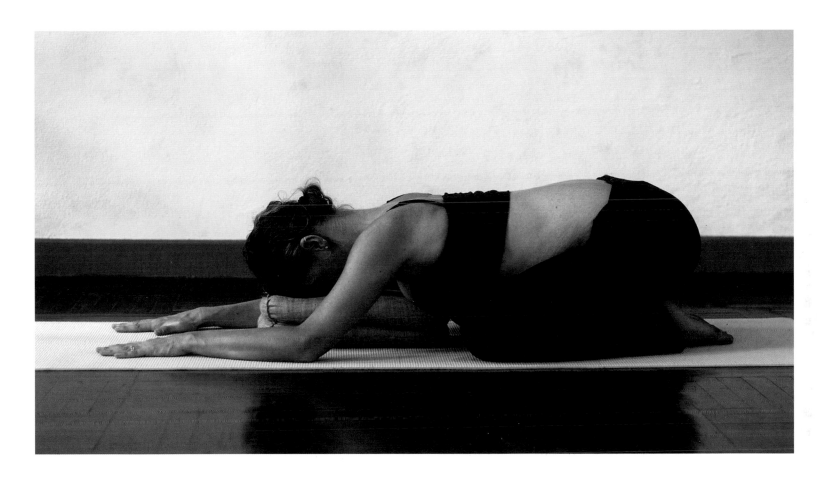

Reflection

By creating a journal of my pregnancy
I have a beautiful keepsake.

NAMASTÉ

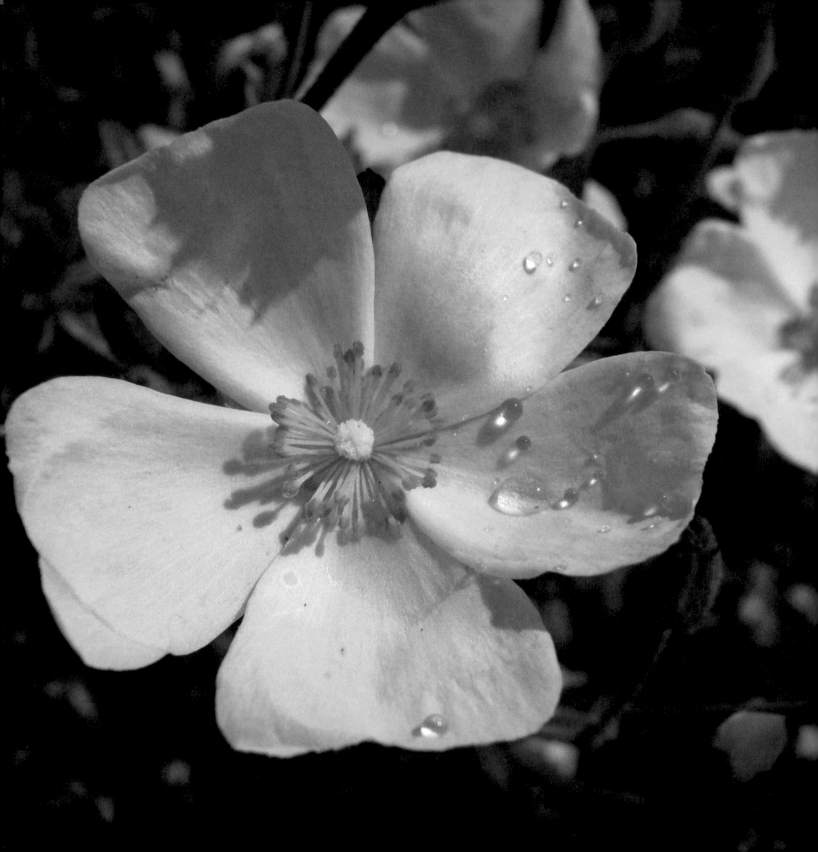

WEEK 38

Transitions

*Giving birth is a natural process and my body is perfectly designed
to do it.*

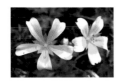

During labor it is important that I remain active, moving my body, focusing on my breath and listening to my instincts so I can remain in control during any transitions.

Although you are full-term you continue to accumulate layers of fat to keep you healthy and snug. Out of sympathy my belly enlarges, my womb full to what feels like capacity as I carry you for these final days.

Despite feeling increasingly uncomfortable and less agile, I practise patience. Soothing my itching belly with aloe vera and massaging my perineum with natural oil to gently stretch it, I prepare for you to arrive and cherish all the wonderful sensations of carrying you inside me for these last remaining days.

My mind is preoccupied with dreams of your birth-day.

I try to dispel any lingering feelings of apprehension and let my anxieties, fears and concerns fade away as the sheer excitement of finally welcoming you into the world and holding you in my arms overwhelms me.

My bag is now packed with all the necessary and personal items I may need for your special day, along with positive thoughts and qualities of courage, faith, patience and acceptance.

BENEFITS: *These Pelvic Rotations can be used during early labor to help keep me active during the surges and encourage you to move down the birth canal, aiding an easier delivery. I can rest in Child's Pose in between surges, offering me respite and an opportunity to gather strength and resilience ready for the rising of the next surge.*

CAUTIONS: *If I have pelvic girdle discomfort or I find this posture uncomfortable I will come on to all fours into a tabletop position and use a birthing ball or the seat of a chair to rest my arms and head on.*

MODIFICATIONS: *I can practise this pose leaning on a bed, seat of a chair, wall or birthing ball.*

Intention

As I arrange all the things we may need for your arrival,
I begin to see my world from a different perspective,
how my life is shifting and changing course as I become
your mother.

Asana for the Week

Tabletop Pelvic Rotations

For this pose I will need a yoga mat.

    This pose is suitable for all stages of my pregnancy.

❁ I come on to all fours into a tabletop position, with my knees slightly wider than my hips (a). Slowly I begin to make small circular movements with my hips, rotating them in a clockwise direction (b). Intuitively I bring my weight forward and back, gradually increasing the size of the circles.

❁ I let my body lead me.

❁ I imagine the rising of a surge ascending through my body.

❁ I notice how my circles become bigger, opening my hips and creating space for you to descend down the birth canal.

❁ As I spiral my hips I visualize you spiraling your body as you pass through my pelvis.

❁ Mindfully I repeat this week's affirmation:

    Giving birth is a natural process and my body is perfectly designed to do it.

❁ As the surge subsides I rest in Child's Pose (c). Resting in this pose gives me time to recover my energy and gather my strength for the next surge.

❁ Here it comes. I feel it rising, engulfing my body, as you continue to make your way through my body. I rise, return to tabletop position and circulate my hips in an anticlockwise direction.

❁ I repeat the above sequence, incorporating first the sound "ooo" as I exhale through my mouth and then the sound "aaahhh."

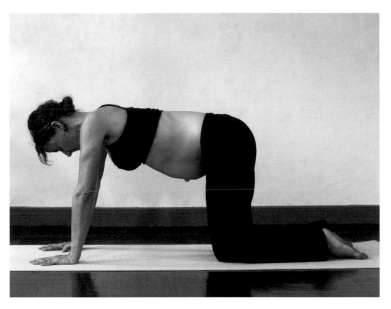

a

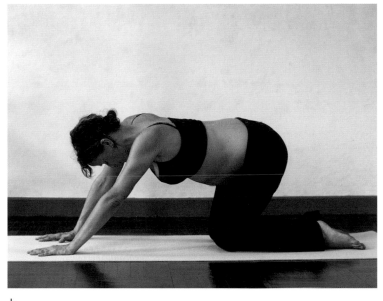

b

Reflection

> *By combining sound with movement and prac-*
> *tising using my breath to release tension and*
> *ease discomfort, I have learnt some valuable*
> *techniques to help me in the early stages of labor*
> *and during the transitions.*
>
> NAMASTÉ

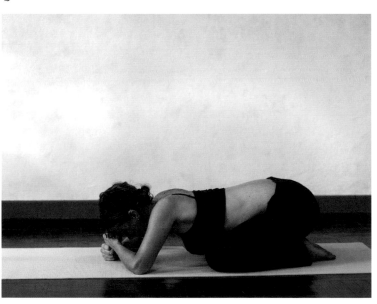

c

WEEK 39

A Labor of Love

*I use my breath to birth my baby;
with each inhalation I gather strength,
with each exhalation I breathe my baby out.*

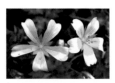

By learning to focus my mind, use my breath and affirm my birth-day wishes, I will affirm my intention of having a labor of love.

I feel you bearing down in my pelvis in readiness for your birth-day. This makes me a little more uncomfortable when I walk and sometimes I find myself literally carrying you to give support and relief to my lower abdomen.

My pelvic area is aching and the gentle squeezes of the Braxton Hicks contractions across my abdomen intensify, training my body for labor.

At times I find myself counting these surges to determine whether they are just pre-labor pains or signs of genuine labor.

I am trying not to become too fixated on the calendar, since I know not many women actually give birth on their predicted due date.

Instead I try to remain flexible in my thoughts, and surrender to the knowledge that I will most likely be taken by surprise, since only you know when you'll be ready to enter this world.

When you do choose to arrive, I am mindful of the fact that you will be moving into a new world with changing sensory stimulation, temperatures, sounds and bright lights. To ease your transition, I will dim the lights, play soothing music and we will cuddle skin-to-skin, so you can nuzzle into my chest, become familiar with my distinctive smell, and find your way to feed from me.

Intention

This week I shall make myself some raspberry leaf tea,
an ideal tincture during these later stages of pregnancy to help prepare
the muscles of my uterus for your birth-day.
With each sip of tea, I will relax and remind myself that
women all over the world give birth to healthy, happy babies,
that our bodies are designed to give birth,
and that my body and my baby know exactly what to do.

Pranayama for the Week

A Breath for Labor

For this pose I will need a yoga mat, a wall and several small cushions.
   This breath is suitable for all stages of my pregnancy.

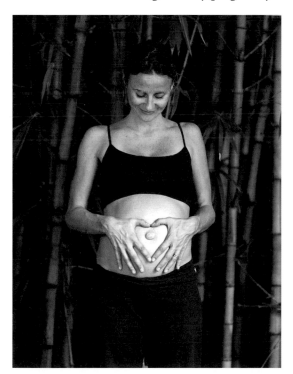

BENEFITS: *A Breath for Labor helps soothe the nervous system; focuses and calms the mind; improves concentration and helps balance emotions.*
A Breath for Labor is a useful breathing technique to use in labor, to help ease discomfort and focus the mind.

MODIFICATIONS: *I will practise using A Breath for Labor in the sequence described in week 38, see pages 132/133.*

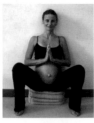

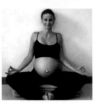

✤ I will choose to sit either in the Supported Squat from Week 12 (see page 40) or Baddha Konasana from week 28 to practise the Birthing Breath described in week 18 (see pages 63/64).

✤ I breathe in through my nose, then parting my lips and teeth slightly I breathe a slow steady breath out through my mouth. I practise this for a few breaths as I close my eyes and day-dream of your birth-day.

✤ In my mind's eye I sense a surge arising.

✤ I begin to breathe A Breath for Labor, rapidly breathing in and out through my mouth for several breaths.

✤ I ride the peak of the surge with my breath. As it begins to subside I fully exhale through my mouth and return to the Birthing Breath, inhaling through my nose and exhaling through my mouth.

✤ I practise this breath for several minutes, then slowly allow my breath to return to its natural pace.

✤ Practising A Breath for Labor three times, I mindfully repeat this week's affirmation:

I use my breath to birth my baby; with each inhalation I gather strength,
with each exhalation I breathe my baby out.

Reflection

Throughout my pregnancy I have united with my baby through my mind, body and breath, practising techniques that will serve and support me to birth my baby in a labor of love.

NAMASTÉ

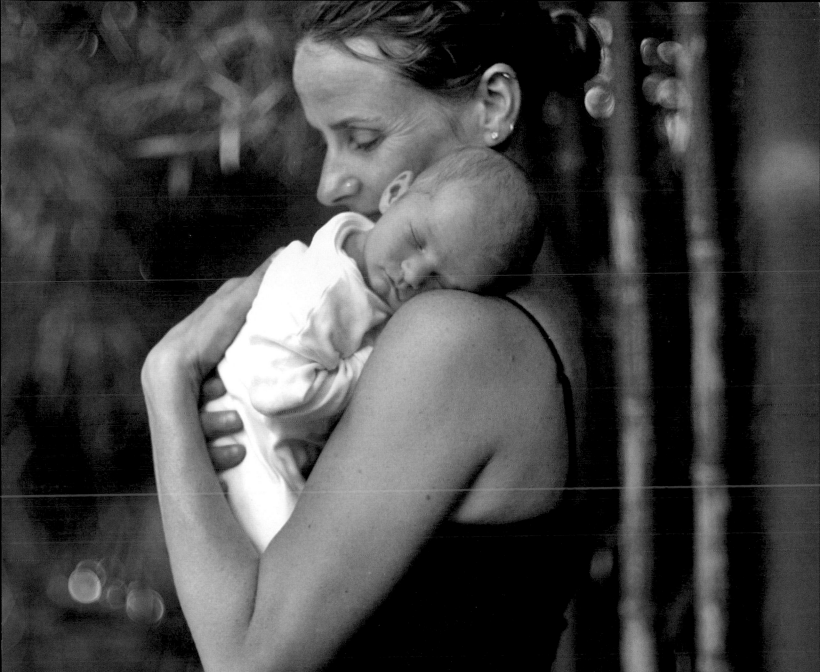

WEEK 40

Happy Birth-Day

I love my baby, my baby loves me.

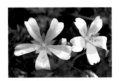

I welcome my new baby into the world with a very **happy birth-day.**

Together we have reached the pinnacle of your incredible journey to life.

Soon you will send a message to my body to release the hormones, to start the birthing process, and my body will escort you down the birth canal. I will be waiting to welcome you into the world.

As my body continues to practise for your birth-day, I am focusing on using my breath and relaxation techniques, which will help support me through the surges when you decide that it is time for you to arrive.

For the last forty weeks my body has been your home, providing you with food, shelter and protection, keeping you warm and snug in your very own uterine world.

Before long you will be entering a very different world.

Even if you choose not to be born this week, I know that we shall meet very soon; it's just a matter of time.

My bag is packed, my birthing intentions visualized, and my heart, bursting with love, is awaits you.

Intention

*This week I shall remember the bag I packed nine months ago.
I will give thanks for all the gifts I have received along the way:
courage, faith, patience, love, laughter, joy, wisdom and strength;
carefully unpacking each one, as I become your mother.*

*BENEFITS: Savasana helps soothe
the nervous system; focuses and
calms the mind; relaxes the
physical body and helps balance
emotions.*

Asana for the Week

Savasana

The final relaxation and a guided visualization. For this pose I will need a yoga mat, a wall
and several small cushions.

This pose and guided relaxation are suitable for all stages of my pregnancy.

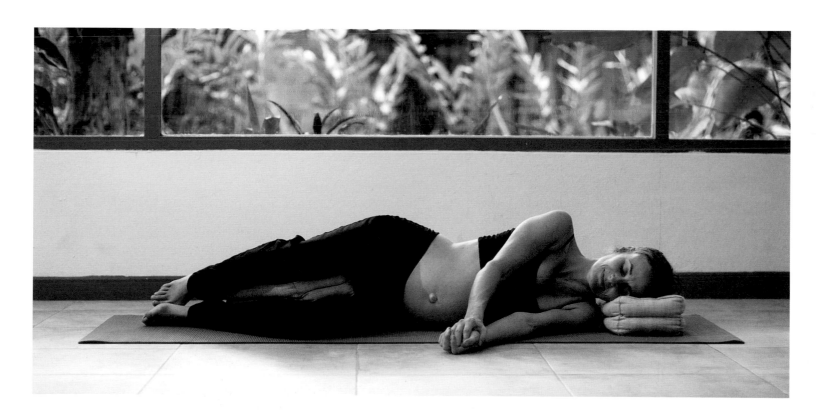

❁ I come to relax in Savasana. I lie on my left side cuddling you.

❁ I make room for you and use several cushions to ensure that we are both comfortable to rest here for up to fifteen minutes. I place a cushion between my thighs and one underneath my belly for you. I rest my head on a cushion.

❁ I close my eyes and breathe.

❁ When I inhale, I breathe in softness, and when I exhale I breathe out any worries or fears [I pause here].

❁ I relax my body [pause]. I relax my thoughts [pause]. I relax my feelings [I take a longer pause here].

❁ Cradling you in my right hand [pause], I bring my awareness into my heart center. I visualize a golden light shining from my heart [pause]. I watch this golden light beam out in all directions, in all dimensions, touching every single cell of my being [pause]. I feel my entire body being bathed in this light, from the soles of my feet to the tips of my fingers and the crown of my head [longer pause].

❁ I see this golden light flowing from my heart center to you.

❁ Mindfully I repeat this week's affirmation:

I love my baby, my baby loves me.

❁ I follow the golden light, watching it pour from my heart into you [pause]. I watch you bathe in this shining light, rolling, tumbling and immersing yourself in the warm glow from my heart [longer pause].

❁ I see this light as a shining sun [pause]. I take my awareness to my cervix, imagining my cervix as a beautiful flower bud waiting to unfurl in the light [pause]. I see each petal of this flower slowly open out in the warmth of this sun [pause].

❁ I imagine you slowly beginning your journey down the birth canal, as the petals of my flower unfold [longer pause].

❁ Mindfully I repeat the affirmation:

When I smile my pelvic-floor muscles smile with me.

- Sensing the gentle pressure of your head crowning, I relax with each breath, using my breath to breathe you out [pause].

- Mindfully I repeat the affirmation:

  I use my breath to birth my baby; with each inhalation I gather strength, with each exhalation I breathe my baby out. [longer pause]

- I watch the golden light beam out as you are born, happy, healthy and shrouded in the warmth of my love. I hold you on my chest; I say to you,

  I love my baby, my baby loves me. [longer pause]

- We are united.

- Slowly I bring my awareness back to my breath, deepening my inhalations and lengthening my inhalations [pause].

- I bring my awareness back into the present moment.

- I unite with you through my mind, body and breath.

- I stay here for a few minutes before using my hands to gently assist me up into a sitting position.

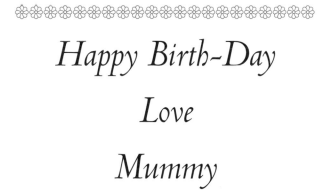

Happy Birth-Day

Love

Mummy

x x x

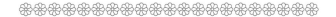

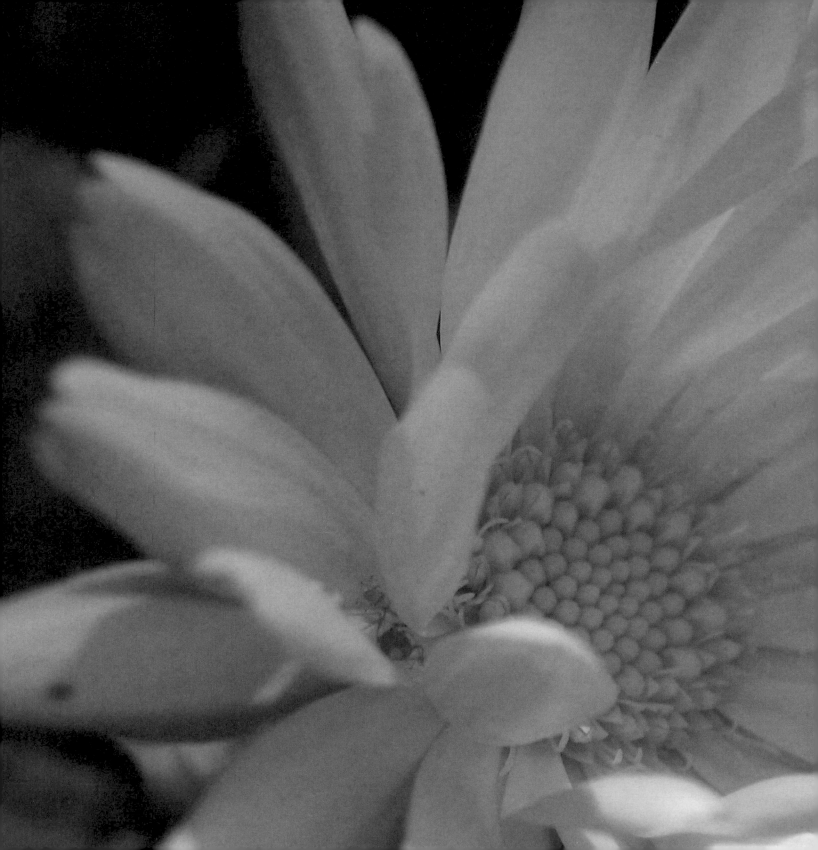

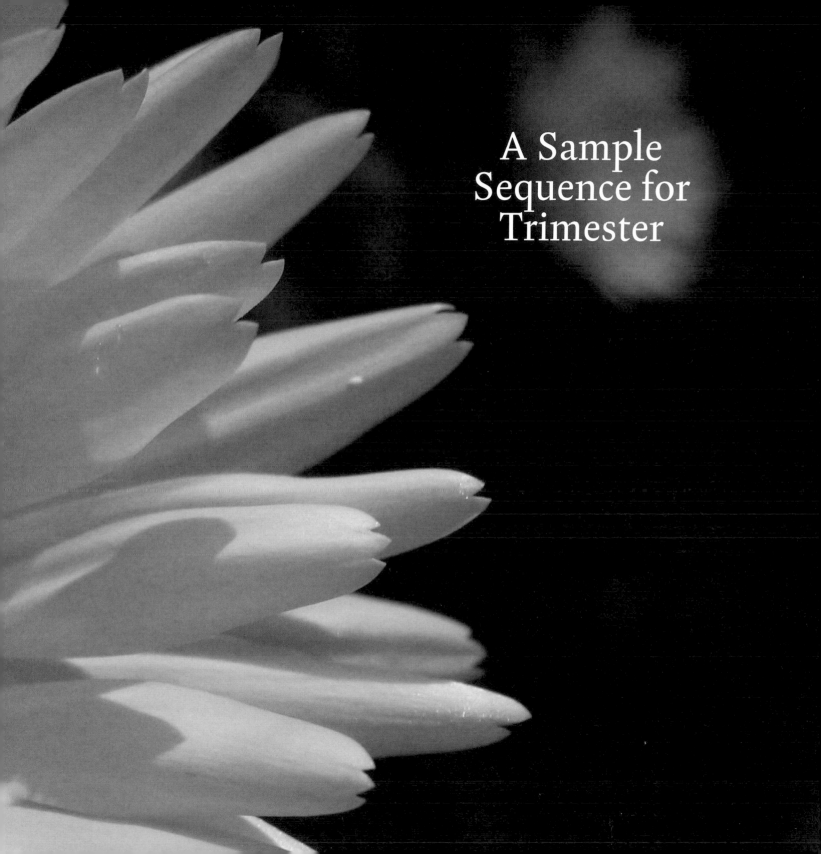

A Sample
Sequence for
Trimester

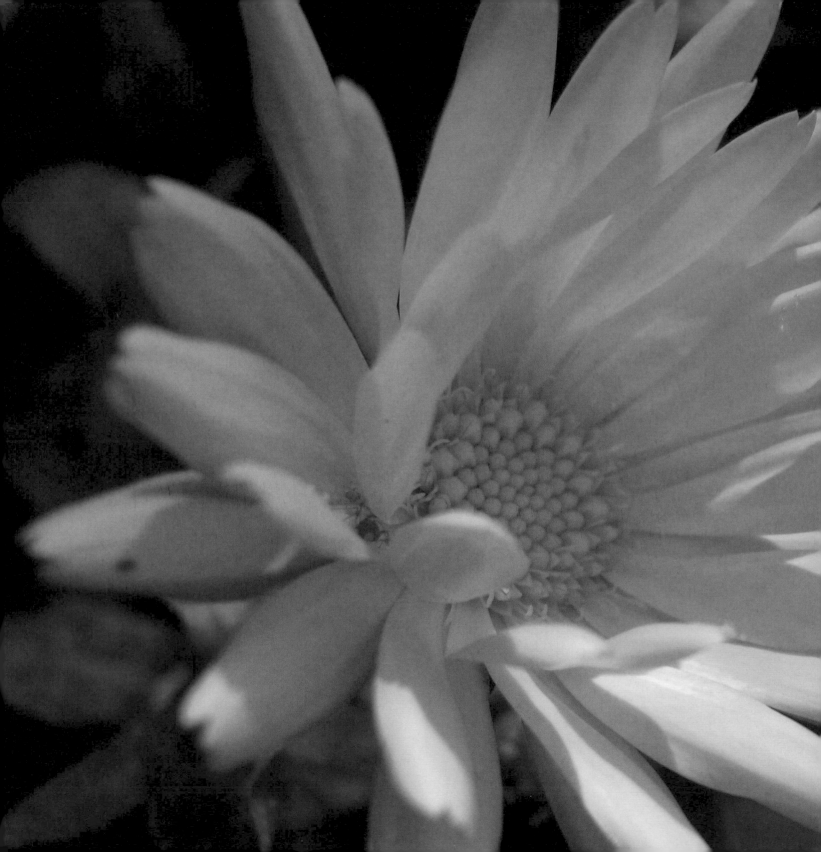

A Sample Sequence for the First Trimester

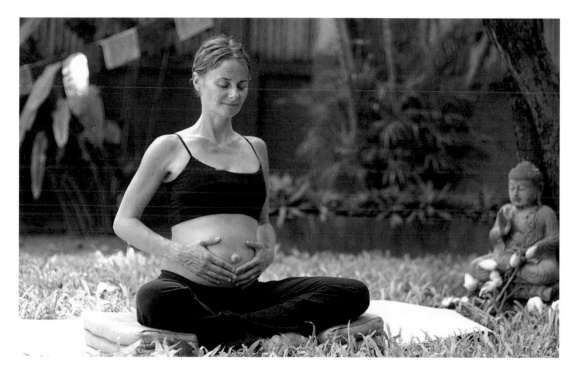

1 Abdominal Breathing

Page 21

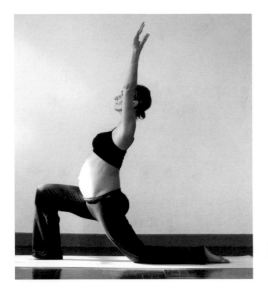

**2 Anjaneyasana –
Crescent Moon**

Pages 90–1

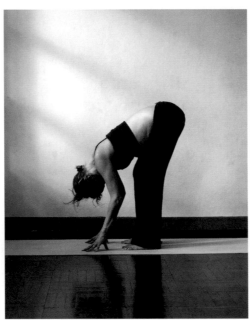

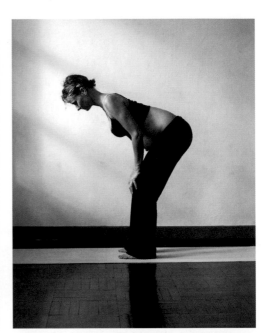

**3 Uttanasana –
Standing Forward Fold**

Pages 32–3

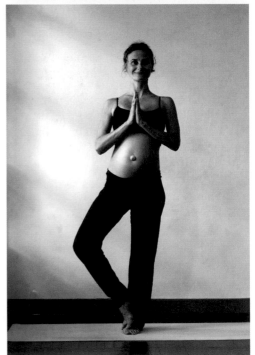

4 Vrksasana – Tree Pose

Pages 36–7

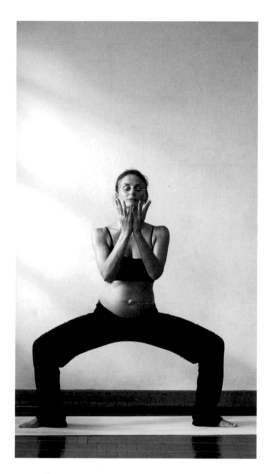
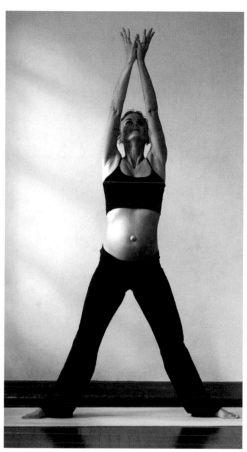
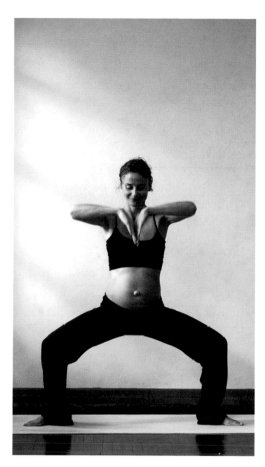

5 Utkata Konasana Flow –
The Goddess Flow

Pages 26–7

6 Parivrtta Sukhasana – Revolved Easy Twist

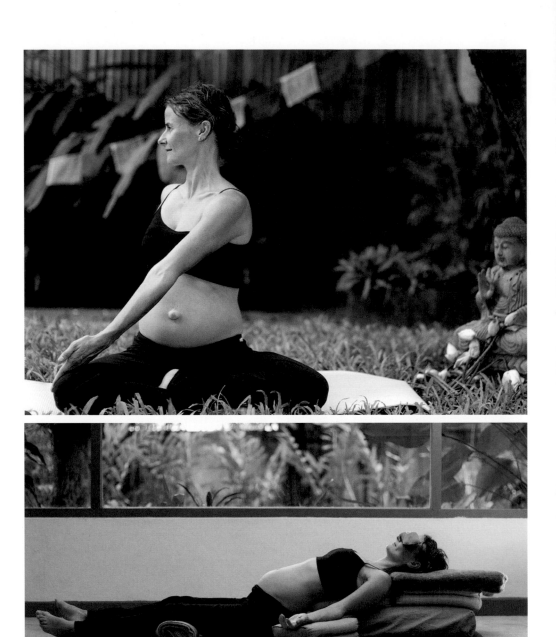

7 Supported Reclining Pose

A Sample Sequence for the Second Trimester

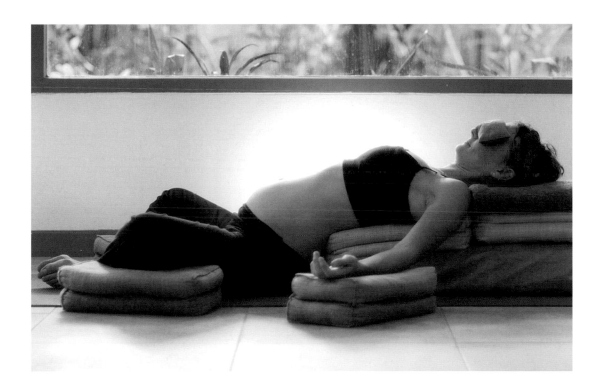

1 Supta Baddha Konasana – Reclined Bound Angle Pose

Pages 122–3

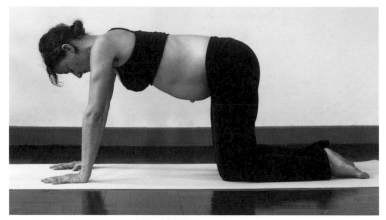

a

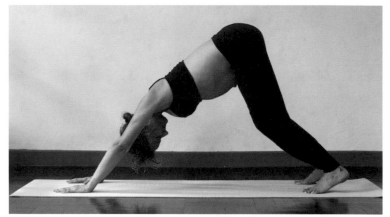

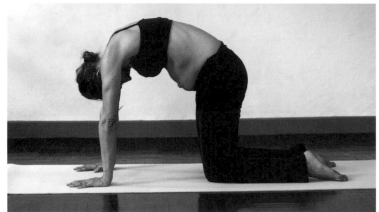

b

2 Cat Sequence

Pages 56–7

Practise the Birthing Breath (see pages 63–4) with the movements.

3 Adho Mukha Svanasana – Downward Facing Dog

Pages 66–7

4 Virabhadrasana I – Warrior 1

Pages 72–3

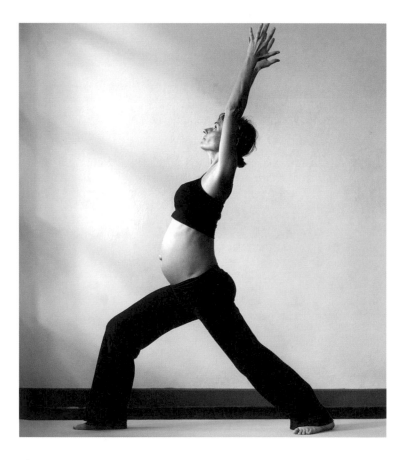

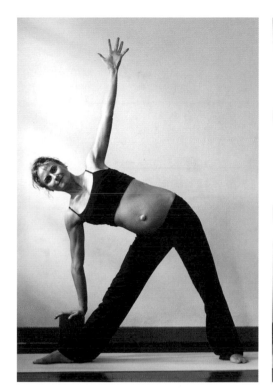

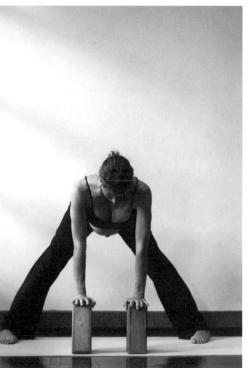

a

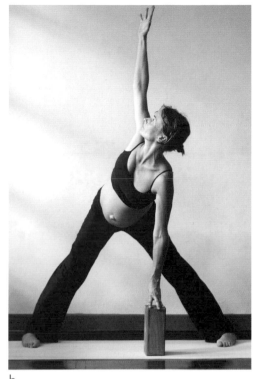

b

5 Trikonasana – Triangle Pose

Pages 82–3

6 Prasarita Padottanasana – Wide Angle Forward Bend with an Open Twist

Pages 46–7

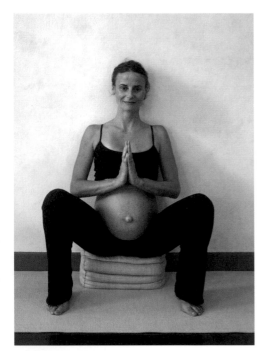

**7 Kegel Exercises –
Pelvic Floor Exercises**

Pages 40–1

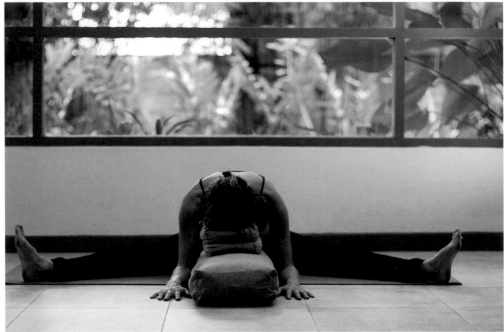

**8 Supported Upavista
Konasana – Supported Wide
Legged Forward Fold**

Pages 96–7

A Sample Sequence for the Third Trimester

1 Baddha Konasana – Bound Angle Pose

Pages 99–100

Practise A Breath for Labor, 135–6

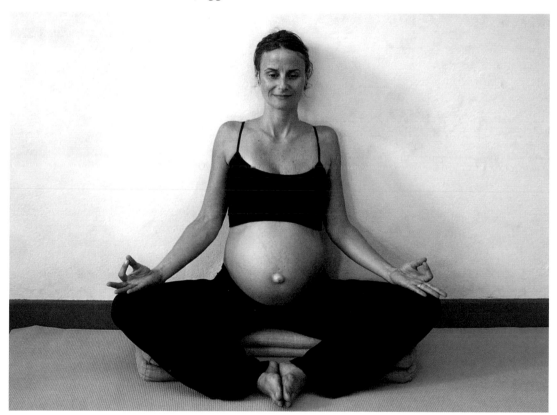

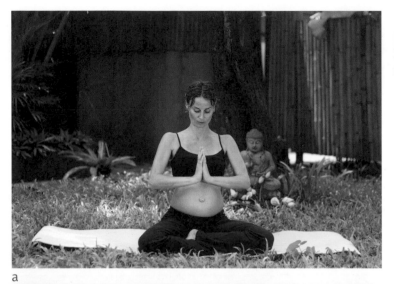

a

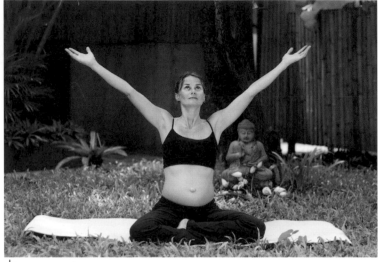

b

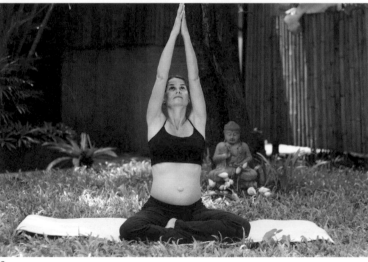

c

2 Seated Namasté Flow

Pages 125–6

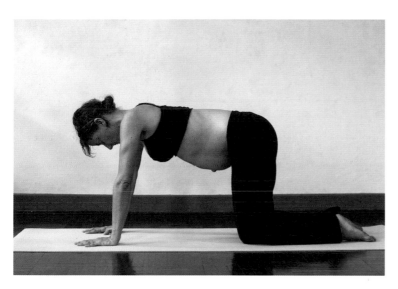

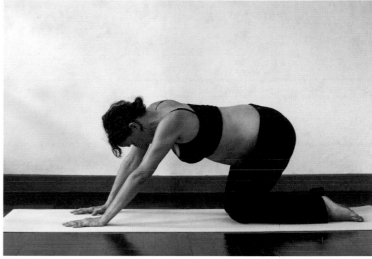

3 Tabletop Pelvic Rotations

Pages 132–3

Practise the Birthing Breath (pages 63–4) with the movements.

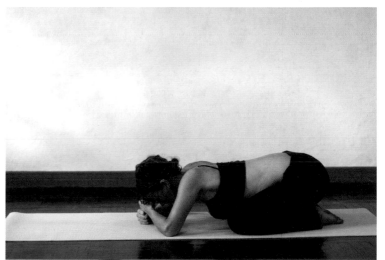

Balasana – Child's Pose

Pages 128–9

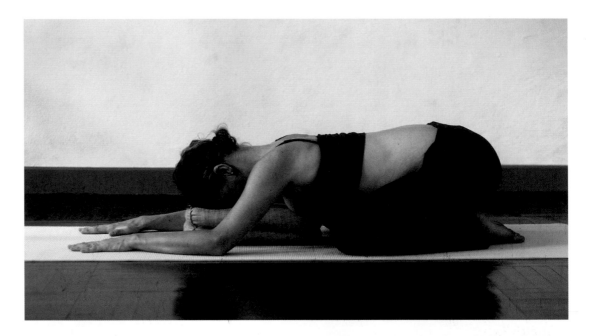

5 Savasana – Relaxation and Visualization

Pages 139–140

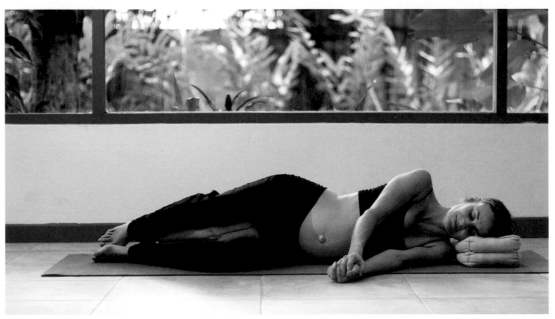

Index of Practices

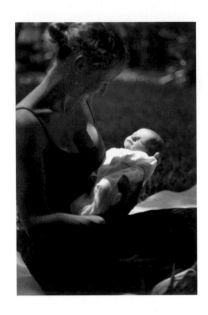

*The light within me bows
to and honors the light
within you.*

                Namasté

About the Author

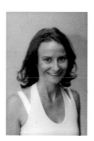

Mel Campbell is a yoga teacher and a mother to three daughters. She was first introduced to the profound benefits of prenatal yoga when she was pregnant with her first child, over thirteen years ago. A dedicated practitioner, she became a certified teacher seven years ago and now teaches adult and children's yoga and prenatal yoga.

Mel has practised prenatal yoga throughout each of her pregnancies. She believes that by nourishing and nurturing body and mind through the practice of yoga mothers to be can keep themselves active and supple and address common pregnancy symptoms, while also preparing the mind, body and spirit for all stages of pregnancy, the birth of their new child and the role of motherhood.

The Yoga of Pregnancy is Mel's first book, and it brings together her two deepest passions: yoga and motherhood. Mel became inspired to write the book when she was pregnant with her third child, Evi, after seeking to draw all the elements of meditation, affirmation and yoga into a practice that deepened her relationship with her growing baby.

She believes that giving birth can be a spiritual experience if we can learn to listen to our instincts, trust, have faith and surrender to the occasion, something that the practice of yoga and meditation during pregnancy can help with.

Mel has travelled the world and pioneered prenatal yoga to Chiang Mai in northern Thailand. Mel is based in the UK, where she shares the wisdom of her studies, experiences and understanding to women, leading yoga of pregnancy classes, workshops and retreats.

For more info about yoga classes with Mel visit www.yogawithmelcampbell.com and www.the-yoga-of-pregnancy.com.

FINDHORN PRESS

Life-Changing Books

For a complete catalogue,
please contact:

Findhorn Press Ltd
117-121 High Street,
Forres IV36 1AB,
Scotland, UK

t +44 (0)1309 690582
f +44 (0)131 777 2711
e info@findhornpress.com

or consult our catalogue online
(with secure order facility) on
www.findhornpress.com

For information on the Findhorn Foundation:
www.findhorn.org